EDITION

Institutional Review Board

MEMBER HANDBOOK

Robert Amdur, MD

Professor of Radiation Oncology
University of Florida
College of Medicine
Gainesville, Florida

Elizabeth A. Bankert, MA

Assistant Provost
Dartmouth College
Hanover, New Hampshire

JONES AND BARTLETT PUBLISHERS
Sudbury, Massachusetts
BOSTON   TORONTO   LONDON   SINGAPORE

World Headquarters

Jones and Bartlett
 Publishers
40 Tall Pine Drive
Sudbury, MA 01776
978-443-5000
info@jbpub.com
www.jbpub.com

Jones and Bartlett
 Publishers Canada
6339 Ormindale Way
Mississauga, Ontario
L5V 1J2
Canada

Jones and Bartlett
 Publishers International
Barb House, Barb Mews
London W6 7PA
United Kingdom

Jones and Bartlett's books and products are available through most bookstores and on-line booksellers. To contact Jones and Bartlett Publishers directly, call 800-832-0034, fax 978-443-8000, or visit our website, www.jbpub.com.

Substantial discounts on bulk quantities of Jones and Bartlett's publications are available to corporations, professional associations, and other qualified organizations. For details and specific discount information, contact the special sales department at Jones and Bartlett via the above contact information or send an email to specialsales@jbpub.com.

Production Credits

Publisher: Kevin Sullivan
Acquisitions Editor: Amy Sibley
Associate Editor: Patricia Donnelly
Editorial Assistant: Rachel Shuster
Associate Production Editor:
 Katie Spiegel
Marketing Manager: Rebecca Wasley

V.P., Manufacturing and Inventory Control:
 Therese Connell
Composition: Auburn Associates, Inc.
Cover Design: Scott Moden
Cover Image: © mmaxer/ShutterStock, Inc.
Printing and Binding: Malloy, Inc.
Cover Printing: Malloy, Inc.

Library of Congress Cataloging-in-Publication Data
Amdur, Robert J.
  Institutional review board : member handbook / Robert Amdur, Elizabeth A. Bankert. — 3rd ed.
    p. ; cm.
  Rev. ed. of: Institutional review board member handbook / Robert J. Amdur, Elizabeth A. Bankert. 2nd ed. c2007.
  Includes bibliographical references and index.
  ISBN 978-0-7637-8000-5
  1. Institutional review boards (Medicine)—Handbooks, manuals, etc. I. Bankert, Elizabeth A. II. Amdur, Robert J. Institutional review board member handbook. III. Title.
  [DNLM: 1. Biomedical Research—ethics—Handbooks. 2. Ethics Committees, Research—organization & administration—Handbooks. 3. Ethical Review—standards—Handbooks. 4. Ethics, Medical—Handbooks. 5. Human Experimentation—ethics—Handbooks. W 20.5 A497i 2011]
  R852.5.A463 2011
  610.68—dc22
                                                            2009054075
6048
Printed in the United States of America
14 13 12 11 10   10 9 8 7 6 5 4 3 2 1

Dedication

This handbook is dedicated to IRB members who understand that protecting the rights and welfare of research subjects requires the motivation to understand complex issues, a commitment to higher ideals, and the courage to make difficult decisions.

> *"Let us all remember that a slower progress in the conquest of disease would not threaten society, grievous as it is to those who deplore that particular disease be not yet conquered, but that society would indeed be threatened by the erosion of those moral values whose loss, possibly caused by too ruthless a pursuit of scientific progress, would make its most dazzling triumphs not worth having."**

---

*Jonas H. 1970. "Philosophical Reflections on Experimenting with Human Subjects." In *Experimentation with Human Subjects*, edited by Paul A. Freund. New York: George Braziller, pp. 16–17.

Contents

Introduction

Congratulations on your membership on the institutional review board (IRB). Service on the IRB is one of the best forms of continuing education available to a person who is interested in medicine or the social sciences because it exposes you to new ideas in a wide range of scientific fields. The decisions you make and the opinions you bring to the IRB will have implications for the people who conduct and participate in research activities.

As an IRB member your mission is to help researchers conduct important studies in a way that protects the rights and welfare of the research participants. People who do not understand how the IRB should function think that making IRB determinations is a simple job that requires little more than common sense and good intentions. This is often not the case. As you learn more about research ethics and research regulation you will understand that many research projects present ethical issues that are not straightforward to recognize or resolve. Common sense and good intentions are required for you to function effectively on the IRB, but these qualities are not enough. You also need a structured approach to evaluating the ethics of a research protocol and a clear understanding of the fundamental principles that you should use to determine how to vote on specific studies. The purpose of this handbook is to provide you with some of the information you need to function optimally as an IRB member.

The first edition of this handbook was published in 2003. Since then we have received feedback on the value of the handbook to IRB members. In response to this feedback, we revised or deleted the chapters that were not helpful and added chapters that address new issues. In this edition we have included chapters to describe IRB review options and discuss IRB member conflict of interest issues. We hope that the third edition of this handbook will help you meet the challenges of IRB work with excitement, enthusiasm, and the tools you need to protect research subjects.

Contributors

Joseph S. Brown, PhD
Professor and Vice-Chair
Department of Psychology
University of Nebraska at Omaha
Omaha, NE

Marianne M. Elliot, MS, CIP
Department of the Navy
Human Research Protection Program
United States Navy
Washington, DC

Dean R. Gallant, AB
Director, Science Center
Executive Officer, Committee on the Use of Human
  Subjects in Research
Harvard University
Cambridge, MA

Bruce G. Gordon, MD, FAAP
Chairman, UNMC Institutional Review Board
Chairman, Joint Pediatric Institutional Review Board
Professor, Pediatric Hematology/Oncology & Stem Cell
  Transplantation
University of Nebraska Medical Center
Omaha, NE

Rachel Homer, BS
Children's Hospital Boston
Boston, MA

Jay G. Hull, PhD
Professor
Psychological and Brain Sciences
Dartmouth College
Hanover, NH

Thomas G. Keens, MD, CIP
Chair, Committee on Clinical Investigations (IRB)
Childrens Hospital Los Angeles
Professor of Pediatrics, Physiology, and Biophysics
Keck School of Medicine of the University of Southern
  California
Los Angeles, CA

Sarah Khan
Medical IRB 2
Office for the Protection of Research Subjects
University of California, Los Angeles
Los Angeles, CA

Susan Z. Kornetsky, MPH, CIP
Director
Clinical Research Compliance
Children's Hospital Boston
Boston, MA

Gail D. Kotulak, BS
IRB Administrator
University of Nebraska Medical Center
Omaha, NE

Christopher J. Kratochvil, MD
Vice-Chair, IRB
Assistant Professor, Psychiatry
University of Nebraska Medical Center
Omaha, NE

Rachel Krebs, BS, CIP
Administrative Director
Office for Human Research Participant Program
Boston College
Chestnut Hill, MA

Linda Medwar, BS
Senior IRB Coordinator
Children's Hospital Boston
Boston, MA

Matthew Miller, MD, MPH, ScD
Associate Director
Health Policy and Management
Harvard Injury Control Research Center
Harvard School of Public Health
Brookline, MA

Paul B. Miller, JD, PhD
Assistant Professor
Faculty of Law
Queen's University
Kingston, ON, Canada

Daniel K. Nelson, MS
Associate Professor and Director
Human Research Studies
School of Medicine
The University of North Carolina at Chapel Hill
Chapel Hill, NC

Robert "Skip" Nelson, MD, PhD
Pediatric Ethicist
Office of Pediatric Therapeutics
Office of the Commissioner, Food and Drug
  Administration
Washington, DC

Ernest D. Prentice, PhD
Associate Dean of Research, Professor, Co-Chair, IRB
Associate Vice-Chancellor for Academic Affairs and
  Regulatory Compliance
University of Nebraska Medical Center
Omaha, NE

Thomas Puglisi, PhD
Deputy Chief Officer
Office of Research Oversight
Department of Veterans Affairs
Washington, DC

Michele Russell-Einhorn, JD
Senior Director
Office for Human Research Studies
Dana Farber Cancer Institute
Boston, MA

Laurie B. Slone, PhD
Assistant Professor
Department of Psychiatry
Dartmouth College
Hanover, NH

Charles Weijer, MD, PhD
Professor of Philosophy and Medicine
Canada Research Chair in Bioethics
Director, Joseph L. Rotman Institute of Science and
  Values
Department of Philosophy
University of Western Ontario
London, ON, Canada

PART
1

BACKGROUND
INFORMATION

The Purpose of This Handbook

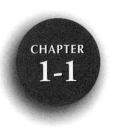

ROBERT AMDUR AND ELIZABETH A. BANKERT

IS THIS HANDBOOK FOR YOU?

This handbook is written specifically for the voting members of an institutional review board (IRB).

WHAT WILL THIS BOOK DO FOR YOU?

This handbook briefly explains the background of the IRB system, what IRB discussions should focus on, and what members should do prior to and during IRB meetings. It also describes the criteria IRB members should use in order to approve a study and summarizes guidelines for evaluating specific types of studies.

WILL THIS HANDBOOK TELL YOU EVERYTHING YOU NEED TO KNOW?

No, this handbook will not tell you everything you need to know about IRBs. This handbook provides basic information that you need to do a thorough job as an IRB member. Frequently you will encounter situations not described in this book. Research ethics and research regulation are complex fields with constantly changing standards and levels of complexity. Continuing education is required to keep up with important IRB issues.

WHAT EDUCATIONAL MATERIALS SHOULD YOU REVIEW IN ADDITION TO THIS HANDBOOK?

There are many publications that explain IRB issues in more detail. Part 4 of this handbook lists additional education resources. We recommend that all IRB members watch the video called *Protecting Human Subjects* that the Office for Human Research Protections (OHRP) will send you for no charge. This video is an excellent review of the history of the IRB system and the fundamental ethical principles that you need to use when evaluating specific research projects. Instructions to order this video can be found on the OHRP website (http://www.hhs.gov/ohrp/). Another resource is a comprehensive textbook on IRB issues called *Institutional Review Board: Management and Function.* We edited this textbook, and many experts in the field of research regulation contributed to it. The target audience for this textbook is IRB administrators and IRB chairs. *Institutional Review Board: Management* and Function can be ordered online at either http://www.jbpub.com or http://www.amazon.com.

Your Mission on the IRB

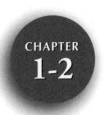

CHAPTER
1-2

ROBERT AMDUR

WHAT IS YOUR ROLE AS AN **IRB** MEMBER?

The mission of the IRB is to protect the rights and welfare of research subjects. This goal should drive every decision that an IRB member makes. A major challenge for IRB members is to avoid getting distracted by issues that are not directly related to the protection of research subjects. To help you focus your efforts when evaluating a research protocol, it will be useful to ask yourself this question:

Is a change in the research protocol likely to improve the welfare of research subjects to a meaningful degree?

If your answer to this question is "no," then you should approve the research proposal without changing it. If your answer to this question is "yes," then you should not approve the research plan as proposed.

WHAT IS AN **IRB**?

The IRB is a committee whose primary responsibility is to protect the rights and welfare of research subjects and to function as a kind of ethics committee focusing on what is right or wrong and on what is desirable or undesirable.

The IRB is an American organization. In other countries, terms such as *Research Ethics Committee* and *Ethical Review Board* are used to describe a committee that evaluates the ethical aspects of research involving human subjects.

There is currently no law or national directive in the United States that requires research to be reviewed in a uniform way regardless of researcher affiliation or funding source. For this reason there are many situations in which research with human subjects is conducted without approval from any type of ethics committee. Similarly, when an organization does set up a system to review the ethics of research protocols, there are many situations in which the review process and approval standards may be customized without regard for external requirements.

In the United States, the only place that an IRB is formally defined is in the code of federal regulations. We will talk briefly about federal regulations later, but at this point it is sufficient to think of the federal regulations as the rules that tell federal agencies and IRBs how they must operate. The criteria for IRB approval according to federal regulations are listed at the end of Chapter 2-7, "Primary Reviewer Presentations," in this book.

Both the U.S. Department of Health and Human Services (HHS) and the Food and Drug Administration (FDA) have regulations that require IRB approval to conduct research that is subject to the authority of these federal agencies. In this setting, the federal regulations present a detailed set of standards that define an IRB and establish the policy and procedures by which an IRB must operate. For the purposes of this handbook, the reference standard for IRB practice is U.S. federal research regulations. This handbook will not discuss alternatives to the federal IRB system.

A Brief History of the IRB System

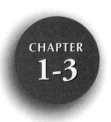

CHAPTER
1-3

ROBERT AMDUR

As recently as 1950, the federal government had a relatively minor role in regulating research conduct. There were no federal regulations that required IRB approval to conduct research involving human subjects, and ethical standards for conducting research were not uniformly applied or accepted.

Today the situation is very different. The federal government now regulates all aspects of the research process through specific agency regulations. The policy and procedures in the federal regulations apply to both biomedical and social science research and define the modern IRB system for monitoring research conduct.

How did we go from so little to so much regulation in a relatively short time? The answer to this question is the history of the modern IRB system. It is a fascinating story that involves the national media, community activism, high-powered science, and big-government politics. A separate book could be written about this subject, but only a cursory review is within the scope of this handbook. The remainder of this chapter will briefly describe the main milestones in the history of research regulation in the United States.

1948: THE NUREMBERG CODE

The Nuremberg trials were conducted at the end of World War II to bring justice to Nazi leaders who had committed crimes against humanity in their treatment of civilian prisoners under their control. A major portion of the trials was devoted to the case of Nazi physicians who had forced prisoners to undergo horrifying procedures for research purposes. To make the case of crimes against humanity, the prosecutors had to argue that the Nazi defendants conducted research in ways that violated the fundamental ethical standards of civilized society. As part of the proceedings at Nuremberg, the prosecution issued what is now referred to as the Nuremberg Code—a document that articulated the basic requirements for conducting research in a way that respects the fundamental rights of research subjects. The full text of the Nuremberg Code can be found on the OHRP website at http://www.hhs.gov/ohrp/references/nurcode.htm. We recommend every IRB member read this document.

The Nuremberg Code explains ethical standards that have been incorporated into most subsequent ethical codes—such as the Declaration of Helsinki—and in federal research regulations. The basic elements of the Nuremberg Code are the requirement for:

- voluntary and informed consent
- a favorable risk/benefit analysis, and
- the right to withdraw without penalty

1955: THE WICHITA JURY STUDY

In the early 1950s, social science researchers at the University of Chicago directed a study to better understand the decision-making process of jurors in criminal trials. A motivation for this study was the concern that showmanship on the part of trial attorneys might have a major influence on the jury verdict. The study involved audio taping jury deliberations in criminal trials in Wichita, Kansas. To avoid influencing their behavior, the jurors were not told that they were subjects of a research project or that their discussions would be recorded.

The investigators completed the study as planned and presented the results in respected academic forums. But public reaction to the Wichita Jury Study was not favorable. The study was criticized in local newspapers, and it soon became the focus of national discussion. The issue was not the details of this particular study but the basic problem of deceiving people for research purposes in a setting where privacy and confidentiality were critically important.

Congressional hearings were held on the subject, and eventually Congress passed a federal law that prohibited the recording of jury deliberations in any setting. There are two main reasons that the events that followed the Wichita study are milestones in the history of research regulation in the United States. These reasons are:

1. The legislation that was passed in response to the Wichita study marks the first time that the actions of well-meaning researchers resulted in the establishment of federal guidelines to protect the public from exploitation.

2. The Wichita study was the first event that focused national attention on the concept that there are settings where important research questions cannot be answered without compromising the integrity of important social institutions. The scientific importance of the Wichita study was never an issue. The rationale for congressional action in this case was that the integrity of the jury process requires an environment where jurors have confidence that an outside party is not observing their deliberations.

1962: THE THALIDOMIDE EXPERIENCE

Thalidomide is a drug that doctors used in the 1950s to treat a variety of unpleasant symptoms associated with pregnancy. At this time, it was not standard practice to inform patients when their doctor was recommending an investigational medication. After treating large numbers of pregnant women with thalidomide, it became clear that this drug caused severe growth deformities in the infants who were exposed to thalidomide in utero. Public outrage over the situation led to an amendment to the Food, Drug, and Cosmetic Act that required investigators to obtain informed consent from potential subjects before administering investigational medications. This legislation is a milestone in the history of research regulation because it was the first time that federal agency regulations were used to establish specific ethical standards for the conduct of research.

1964: NIH ETHICS COMMITTEE

In the mid-1950s, the Clinical Research Center (CRC) at the National Institutes of Health (NIH) was created to oversee the conduct of clinical research. CRC policy required that all research conducted at this facility be approved by a committee focusing on ethical issues. The same process was going on less formally at both public and private institutions all over the country, where local investigators saw the need for a formal review of the ethical implications of research activity. A milestone in the use of ethical review committees came in 1964 when NIH director James Shannon established a policy that required an ethics committee to review all research funded by the Public Health Service. As part of this effort, Dr. Shannon articulated the need for a formal process to ensure that all research involving human subjects be conducted according to a uniform set of ethical standards.

1964: THE WORLD MEDICAL ASSOCIATION DECLARATION OF HELSINKI

In 1964, the World Medical Association met in Helsinki, Finland, to draft the Declaration of Helsinki, a document that would build on the Nuremberg Code of 1948 to describe the standards of ethical research involving human subjects. The association has met many times since 1964 to reaffirm or make minor revisions to the declaration. Last revised in 2000, the Declaration of Helsinki basically consists of the standards described in the Nuremberg

Code plus statements that make the following two key points:

1. That the interests of the subject should always be given a higher priority than those of society

2. That every subject in clinical research should get the best known treatment

1966: THE ETHICS OF CLINICAL RESEARCH AND THE *NEW ENGLAND JOURNAL OF MEDICINE*

In 1966 the *New England Journal of Medicine* published an article entitled "Ethics of Clinical Research," by Henry Beecher, a senior member of the Department of Anesthesiology at Harvard Medical School. In this article, Dr. Beecher described 22 studies that had been conducted by respected investigators and recently published in prestigious medical journals. For each of these studies, Beecher explained why the study was unethical based on fundamental principles such as lack of informed consent and increased risk to subjects. His conclusion about the status of medical research in the United States left no room for misunderstanding:

> What seem to be breaches of ethical conduct in experimentation are by no means rare but are almost, one fears, universal. . . . A particularly pernicious myth is the one that depends on the view that ends justify means. A study is ethical or not at its inception . . . whoever gave the investigator the godlike right of choosing martyrs? (Beecher, 1966)

Beecher's article is a milestone in the history of research ethics because it was an unprecedented attempt by a respected member of the research community to focus attention on the need to improve the ethical standards for conducting clinical research in this country. An article of this length is rarely seen in medical literature today. Although it is not essential that IRB members read this article to function effectively on the IRB, doing so may help give one the confidence and insight that one needs to question accepted research procedures.

1973: CONGRESSIONAL HEARINGS ON THE QUALITY OF HEALTH CARE AND HUMAN EXPERIMENTATION

In 1973, Senator Edward Kennedy directed a series of congressional hearings in response to public concern about ethical problems in the way medical research was being conducted in this country. The main catalyst for conducting these hearings was public reaction to a federally sponsored study on the natural history of syphilis called the Tuskegee syphilis experiment. However, it is more accurate to view this period of congressional activity as the result of a long string of high-profile events involving both biomedical and social science research. The remainder of this section briefly describes some of the events that were pivotal in focusing public attention on issues related to research ethics. The purpose of the remainder of this chapter is to give IRB members a feel for the issues congressional representatives were thinking about when they debated the need for extending federal oversight of research involving human subjects.

Willowbrook Hepatitis Studies

In the 1950s, a series of studies were done to understand issues related to the transmission of the hepatitis virus in retarded children who were residents in the Willowbrook state school, an extended care facility in New York state. Because a high percentage of residents contracted hepatitis during their time at Willowbrook, there was no question about the importance of understanding more about the mode of transmission of the hepatitis virus in this population. The aspect of this research that generated debate in both the national media and professional journals was a study design that involved intentionally infecting healthy children with hepatitis by feeding them a solution made from the feces of children with active hepatitis. Parents were told their child would not be cared for at Willow-brook unless they participated in this study.

Jewish Chronic Disease Hospital Studies

In the 1960s, doctors conducted a series of studies on chronically ill, mostly demented patients in the Jewish Chronic Disease Hospital in New York City. All of the subjects had illnesses that compromised their immune system. The purpose of the research was to determine how a weakened immune system influenced the spread of cancer. To evaluate this issue, doctors injected live cancer cells into the bloodstream of the subjects. Informed consent was not obtained from patients or their families.

Milgram Studies of Obedience to Authority

In the early 1960s, psychologist Stanley Milgram conducted a series of studies that continue to generate controversy. Dr. Milgram designed these studies in the aftermath of World War II when the world was trying to understand the genocide of the Holocaust. The purpose of the Milgram studies was to understand why people follow the directions of authority figures even when they are told to do things that are cruel and unethical.

The experiment involved subjects who were deceived into thinking that they were helping with a study to evaluate the role of negative reinforcement on learning. A study director instructed the study subject to deliver an electric shock when a person who was playing the role of the learner answered a question incorrectly. As the study progressed, the subject was instructed to give progressively stronger punishment shocks. More than half of the subjects eventually delivered what they thought were high-intensity, potentially lethal shocks in spite of expressions of serious distress on the part of the person who was playing the role of the learner. After completion of the study, the subjects were debriefed about the true purpose of the study, the nature of the deception, and potential implications of their behavior. Many of the subjects said that the cruelty of their actions was profoundly upsetting.

San Antonio Contraception Study

In the early 1970s, a study was conducted in a contraception clinic in San Antonio, Texas, that evaluated the efficacy of different kinds of female contraceptive pills. The clinic served predominantly indigent patients who had no other place to go for contraceptive medication. The study randomized subjects between active contraceptive and placebo pills. The women were not informed that they were the subjects of this type of research or that they might be receiving inactive medication. As expected, there were a high number of unplanned pregnancies in the placebo group.

Tearoom Trade Study

In the early 1970s, social scientist Laud Humphries conducted a study of homosexual behavior in public restrooms. Dr. Humphries was able to function as a watch queen outside public restrooms where people gathered to engage in anonymous homosexual activity. Humphries recorded the license numbers and other identifying information from the people who came for these kinds of interactions and used this information to obtain names and addresses. He went to the homes of his study subjects and presented himself as an interviewer to collect information about the subject's background and family life. Many of the subjects were living with their family in a situation where it would be devastating to reveal information about homosexual activity. At no time did the subjects understand that they were participating in research. In published reports of this study, the level of detail revealed the identity of some of the subjects.

Tuskegee Syphilis Study

Between 1932 and 1972, the U.S. Public Health Service funded a study to evaluate the natural history of untreated syphilis in human beings. When this study started, the basic concept was considered scientifically important and ethically justifiable because there was no effective treatment for this devastating disease. In retrospect, the main problem with this research was that the subject population was one of the most vulnerable in our society—

approximately 300 indigent, uneducated, African American sharecroppers in Macon County in Alabama who were living with syphilis. This study is now infamous in the world of research ethics and research regulation. It is usually referred to as the Tuskegee study, the Tuskegee syphilis study, or simply Tuskegee in reference to the city in Alabama where the study was headquartered.

The subjects of the Tuskegee study did not have a meaningful understanding of their condition or the nature of the research in which they were participating. Although deception may not have been intentional on the part of the investigators, the reality is that the subjects thought they were receiving beneficial medical care and did not understand that the purpose of the project was to document the course of their illness without treatment. Tests and procedures—such as spinal taps—were done solely for research purposes. The study doctors followed the subjects without treatment for many years after penicillin became widely available and known to be beneficial in the treatment of syphilis. Public outrage in response to high-profile stories about the exploitation of research subjects forced the investigators to stop the study in 1972.

The fact that the Tuskegee study was directed by the federal government over such a long period of time has stained the integrity of the American research enterprise to a degree that will affect our thinking about research ethics and regulation for years to come. There are articles and books about the ethical implications of the Tuskegee study, and it has become a milestone in the history of research regulation. This study was the main reason that the principle of justice was developed in the Belmont Report. Public reaction to the Tuskegee study also catalyzed a series of events that led to passage of the National Research Act of 1974.

1974: THE NATIONAL RESEARCH ACT AND THE IRB SYSTEM

Following congressional hearings directed by Senator Kennedy in 1973, the basic consensus was that federal oversight was required to protect the rights and welfare of research subjects. It is important to note that public concern was not limited to medical or biomedical research. The Wichita jury study, the Milgram studies, and the Tearoom Trade study are only some of the research activities that led our congressional representatives to conclude that social science research also needed additional regulation.

This chapter began by asking a question: How did we go from almost no federal oversight of research in 1950 to the extensive system of federal laws and regulations that we have today? The short answer is that in 1974, Congress passed the National Research Act in response to a long list of events that convinced the American public that human subjects were being exploited and harmed on a regular basis by both biomedical and social science researchers. The act did two things that have shaped the standards and procedures that we use to regulate research today—it established the modern IRB system and the National Commission for Protection of Human Subjects of Biomedical and Behavioral Research.

The Modern IRB System

The National Research Act of 1974 established the modern IRB system for regulating research involving human subjects. The act passed federal regulations that required IRB approval to conduct most kinds of research involving human subjects, defined the policy and procedures that an IRB must follow when reviewing research, and established the criteria that an IRB must use to approve research conduct.

As mentioned in other sections of this handbook, it is not important for IRB members to focus on the specific regulations and federal agencies that direct IRB policy and procedures. However, some IRB members may find it useful to understand that, as directed by the National Research Act of 1974, the HHS initially promulgated the main IRB regulations in 1981 in Title 45, Part 46 of the Code of Federal Regulations (45 CFR 46). These regulations were revised as recently as November 2001, and additional sections continue to be created in response to new thinking and specialized issues. In 1991, 17 federal agencies adopted HHS regulations at 45 CFR 46. Because these regulations are now common to most federal agencies, the HHS regulations at 45 CFR 46 are referred to as the Common Rule.

It may be confusing to people who are not familiar with the structure of federal agencies, but IRB members may hear discussions in which a distinction is made between the Common Rule or HHS regulations and FDA regulations related to IRB review of research. Although the FDA is actually part of the Department of Health and Human Services, HHS and the FDA have separate regulations related to research involving human subjects. In other words, the FDA has not signed on to the Common Rule. But, because the differences between HHS and FDA regulations related to the IRB are minor, the HHS-FDA differences rarely influence IRB decisions.

The National Commission for the Protection of Human Subjects of Biomedical and Behavioral Research

The National Research Act of 1974 established the National Commission for the Protection of Human Subjects of Biomedical and Behavioral Research. The debates and hearings that led to the National Research Act of 1974 made it clear that establishing ethical standards for the conduct of research was not a simple matter. Although Congress did establish specific research regulations, the legislators involved with this effort recognized that there were many situations where it was difficult to know what to do. To help clarify what should be done in settings that are ethically challenging, the National Research Act of 1974 created a special committee called the National Commission for Protection of Human Subjects of Biomedical and Behavioral Research. Made up of a diverse group of people representing the fields of ethics, religion, law, industry, medicine, and other disciplines, the committee is often referred to as the National Commission.

Between 1975 and 1978, the National Commission issued multiple reports that defined problems and made recommendations regarding the conduct of research in specific populations. For example, the group published reports on research involving children, pregnant women, prisoners, and people with dementia. These population-specific reports were important in establishing the ethical framework that we use today to think about research in vulnerable populations, and in many cases federal regulations and other guidelines were revised in response to the National Commission's recommendations. In 1978, the commission issued the Belmont Report, a major milestone in research ethics and research regulation. The Belmont Report is the subject of the next chapter.

REFERENCE

Beecher, H. (1966). Ethics of clinical research. *New England Journal of Medicine, 274*, 1354–1360.

Principles of the Belmont Report

ROBERT AMDUR

Ethical Principles of the Belmont Report

PRINCIPLE 1: RESPECT FOR PERSONS

- Treat individuals as autonomous agents.
- Protect persons with diminished autonomy.

PRINCIPLE 2: BENEFICENCE

- Do unto others as you would have them do unto you.

PRINCIPLE 3: JUSTICE

- Distribute the risks and potential benefits of research equally among those who may benefit from the research.

THE NATIONAL COMMISSION AND THE BELMONT REPORT

The National Research Act of 1974 established the National Commission for Protection of Human Subjects of Biomedical and Behavioral Research. This commission was a committee with a goal to clarify the ethical guidelines applying to research involving human subjects in any setting. After issuing a series of reports that discussed research involving especially vulnerable subject populations such as prisoners and children, the commission conducted a series of core meetings related to this work at the Belmont Conference Center near Baltimore, Maryland. The report that the National Commission issued in 1978 to explain the fundamental ethical principles that should guide the conduct of research involving human subjects is called the Belmont Report.

The Belmont Report is an eight-page document that clearly explains the three principles that are the main tools that all IRB members should use to evaluate the ethics of specific research proposals. The Belmont Report is on the OHRP website, which is at http://www.hhs.gov/ohrp/humansubjects/guidance/belmont.htm. The remainder of this chapter will summarize the three ethical principles of the Belmont Report.

BELMONT PRINCIPLE 1: RESPECT FOR PERSONS

The principle of respect for persons incorporates the following two main ethical convictions related to individual autonomy:

1. Individuals are treated as autonomous agents.

2. Persons with diminished autonomy are given protection.

There are four conditions that follow directly from the principle of respect for persons, and these conditions are requirements for IRB approval of research. The conditions are:

1. Voluntary consent to participate in research

2. Informed consent to participate in research

3. Protection of privacy and confidentiality

4. The right to withdraw from research participation without penalty

The Right to Individual Autonomy and Self-Determination

According to the first ethical conviction involving the principle of respect for persons, each individual has the right to autonomy and self-determination. This means that each person has the right to determine his or her own destiny.

The second ethical conviction involving respect for persons involves protection for individuals whose ability to act autonomously is compromised. Children have diminished autonomy because of their intellectual development and legal status in society. Prisoners have diminished autonomy because they have forfeited certain basic personal liberties. People who are in situations that affect their ability to think clearly have compromised autonomy when they cannot understand their situation well enough to control their own destiny. Similarly, people who do not have the educational background to understand the implications of research participation cannot control their own destiny when faced with the decision to participate in a research study.

Vulnerable Subjects

In the language of research regulation, the term *vulnerable* describes a person who is likely to have compromised autonomy related to decisions about research participation to a degree that would violate the principle of respect for persons. To say that subjects are vulnerable means that they are likely to have compromised autonomy to a degree that demands extra protection.

Protecting Vulnerable Subjects

The second main ethical conviction of the principle of respect for persons is that persons with diminished autonomy are entitled to protection to prevent exploitation. In many situations, it is difficult to decide if persons who are likely to have diminished autonomy should be excluded from research. Preventing people from making a decision about research participation may violate the principle of respect for persons because it denies them the right of self-determination. When there are conflicting issues related to respect for persons, the principle itself requires judgment decisions that evaluate potential risks and benefits for specific subjects.

In addition to excluding people with compromised autonomy, there are many things that researchers and the IRB can do to increase the protection of vulnerable subjects. For example, when subjects are incapacitated, the research plan could require informed consent from a well-educated and properly motivated surrogate decision maker. When the potential for coercion is high, the research plan could require that an independent subject advocate monitor the consent process. When comprehension of important information is the issue, the research plan could include provisions to test the subject's understanding of the important information prior to enrollment.

Coercion or Undue Influence Versus Voluntary Actions

In order to implement the Belmont principle of respect for persons, it is important to understand the concept of *coercion*. Coercion means that a person is to some degree forced, or at least strongly pushed, to do something that is not good for him to do. In discussions of research regulation, the term *undue influence* is often used to describe the concept of coercion.

Coercion is a concept that is impossible to define beyond a certain point. Like pornography, it is difficult to define, but you know it when you see it. Does your salary coerce you into going to work? If you say no, then consider whether you would quit if you didn't get paid. The point is that it is not possible to define coercion in a way that establishes a clear line between situations that are, and are not, ethical.

Coercion is unethical because individuals who are coerced into participating in research have diminished autonomy—meaning they do not have the ability to control their own destiny. Said another way, if individuals are put in a position where there is undue influence to participate in research, then their ability to control their own destiny has been compromised. The term that is used to explain the situation where there is no significant coercion or undue influence is *voluntary*. The principle of respect for persons requires that decisions regarding research participation be made voluntarily, without coercion or undue influence.

Informed Consent

A fundamental issue for the conduct of ethical research is the concept of *informed consent*. Informed consent means that subjects understand the important implications of the decision to participate in research, and they actively agree to such participation. Informed consent is a condition that follows directly from the principle of respect for persons.

The conduct of research with subjects who are not competent to give informed consent is one of the most controversial issues in research ethics. Conducting research based on permission from someone other than the research subject is based on the concept of *substituted judgment*, which basically means that the person making the decision knows what the subject would want to do in that situation. Obviously, such assumptions are fraught with problems. It is for this reason that people who are not capable of making informed decisions are described as "vulnerable," and the principle of respect for persons requires that they be given protection so that their right to individual autonomy is preserved to an acceptable degree.

Privacy and Confidentiality

The protection of privacy and confidentiality is a concept that follows directly from the principle of respect for persons. For most IRB members, it will be useful to think of privacy and confidentiality as they relate to potentially damaging or embarrassing information about a research subject. The 1993 Office for Human Research Protections *IRB Guidebook* defines privacy as "having control over the extent, timing, and circumstances of sharing oneself (physically, behaviorally, or intellectually) with others" (OHRP, 1993, Chapter III) and that confidentiality "pertains to the treatment of information that an individual has disclosed in a relationship of trust and with the expectation that it will not be divulged to others in ways that are inconsistent with the understanding of the original disclosure without permission" (OHRP, 1993, Chapter III).

Privacy and confidentiality are actions that follow from the principle of respect for persons and individual autonomy. Such concepts allow research subjects to control who has access to information that may harm them. The harm that results from invasion of privacy or breach in confidentiality is usually social harm because it compromises a person's reputation, financial status, employability, or insurability, or in some way results in stigmatization or discrimination.

BELMONT PRINCIPLE 2: BENEFICENCE

The Belmont Report describes the principle of beneficence as being an obligation to secure the well-being of the research subject. Some people think that beneficence is just another way of emphasizing the rule of "do no harm." From the standpoint of making IRB determinations, it is probably better to think of this principle as a commitment that goes beyond do no harm to include the conviction that research should be designed to maximize potential benefits and minimize potential risks.

Most IRB members will find it useful to translate the term *beneficence* into something more familiar that captures the important aspects of this fundamental ethical principle. Some experienced IRB members prefer to think of beneficence as a requirement to be kind to subjects or to do unto others as you would have them do unto you. IRB members should use these standards when evaluating research proposals. Specifically:

• To determine if a research proposal supports the principle of beneficence, each IRB member should ask the following question: "Are research subjects treated the way that I would like to be treated in this situation?"

The principle of beneficence also requires IRB members to evaluate the risks and potential benefits of research participation.

- The risks of research are justified by the potential benefits to the individual and/or society.
  The IRB is sometimes forced to make a value judgment related to the trade-off between the implications of research for the individual versus those of society. The Belmont Report acknowledges that this is an unavoidable conflict that must be resolved on a case-by-case basis.
- The study is designed so that risks are minimized and potential benefits are maximized.
  This means that the IRB is required to evaluate the quality of the science in a research proposal, the qualifications of the investigator, the resources available to accomplish the study as planned, and the methods used in the study relative to the available alternatives. It is the principle of beneficence that directs the IRB to evaluate fundamental aspects of study design such as the characteristics of the control group and the statistical power calculations.
- Conflicts of interest are managed so that bias in important judgments related to research conduct is unlikely.
  A conflict of interest that is likely to bias important judgments about the conduct of research violates the principle of beneficence because it means that risks to subjects are not minimized.

BELMONT PRINCIPLE 3: JUSTICE

The principle of justice is more difficult to understand and implement than the principles of respect for persons and beneficence because the concept of justice relates to the distribution of risk within society. It may be useful to understand that the Belmont Report defined the principle of justice in response to studies that appeared to exploit some of the most vulnerable segments of our society—such as the Tuskegee syphilis study. As explained in the Belmont Report, the principle of justice says the following:

- The potential risks of research should be borne equally by the members of our society who are likely to benefit from it.
  To apply the principle of justice when evaluating a research proposal, the IRB must evaluate the characteristics of the study population.
- The research project does not systematically select specific classes or types of individuals simply because of their ease of availability or their compromised position as opposed to reasons directly related to the problem being studied.
  The Belmont Report mentions welfare patients, particular racial or ethnic minorities, and persons confined to institutions as examples of classes of subjects that would raise concern based on the principle of justice.

The previous discussion summarizes the principle of justice as the Belmont Report describes it. The traditional application of the principle of justice has focused on which subjects are *included* in research when they should not be. However, in the past 20 years, several activist groups have interpreted the principle of justice to mean that it is unethical to *exclude* classes of people who are likely to benefit from research participation. Specific examples of this interpretation of the principle of justice are the exclusion of women of childbearing potential from Phase 3 investigational drug trials and the exclusion of children from research involving investigational drugs that are primarily used in adults. Both practices are currently being challenged on the grounds that it violates the principle of justice to deny these groups the benefit of knowing how research results apply to them. If one accepts this interpretation of the principle of justice, the principle of justice also requires the following:

- The research project does not systematically exclude a specific class or type of person who is likely to benefit from research participation or in whom the results of a specific kind of research are likely to be applied.

REFERENCE

Office for Human Research Protections (OHRP). (1993). *IRB guidebook.* Washington, DC: U.S. Department of Health and Human Services. Available: http://www.hhs.gov/ohrp/irb /irb_guidebook.htm.

IRB Review Categories

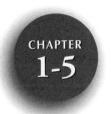

ROBERT AMDUR AND ELIZABETH A. BANKERT

IRB Review Categories

There are three categories of IRB review:

Exempt from further IRB review: A project that is exempt from IRB review does not require further regulatory review, including continuing review.

Expedited review: Expedited review can be carried out by the IRB chairperson or by one or more experienced reviewers. In reviewing the research, the reviewers may exercise all of the authorities of the IRB except that the reviewers may not disapprove the research. The review process involves the same criteria as full-committee review, and continuing review must occur at least on an annual basis after approval.

Full-committee review: The IRB determination requires a majority vote by a quorum of the full IRB committee with continuing review at least annually.

HUMAN SUBJECT, RESEARCH, AND EXEMPT AND EXPEDITED REVIEW CATEGORIES

The primary focus of this handbook is the role of the IRB member at a full-committee meeting. However, it is useful for IRB members to understand that there are projects that the IRB does not have authority to regulate, and other projects that may be handled by the IRB with a process other than a full-committee review.

IRB Purview

Federal regulations give the IRB the authority to review research involving human subjects. IRB authority does not extend to projects that are not research or projects in which the subject of the research is not a human subject. For this reason, the regulatory definitions of *research* and *human subject* are the starting point for determining the role of the IRB in evaluating a project.

Research: a systematic investigation, including research development, testing, and evaluation, designed to develop or contribute to generalizable knowledge.

Human subject: a living individual about whom an investigator (whether professional or student) conducting research obtains (1) data through intervention or interaction with the individual, or (2) identifiable private information.

Once a project is determined to be under the purview of the IRB, the research can be reviewed via three categories, depending on the nature of the research. The categories are exempt, expedited, and full committee. In most cases, the IRB office makes the determination as to which category of review is appropriate.

Projects That May Be Exempt From Further IRB Review

A project that is exempt from IRB review does not require further regulatory review, including continuing review. Most of the projects that may be exempt from further IRB review fall into one of the following three categories:

1. Research conducted in established or commonly accepted educational settings, involving normal educational practices.

2. Research involving the use of educational tests (cognitive, diagnostic, aptitude, achievement), survey procedures, interview procedures, or observation of public behavior, unless: (i) information obtained is recorded in such a manner that human subjects can be identified, directly or through identifiers linked to the subjects; and (ii) any disclosure of the human

subjects' responses outside the research could reasonably place the subjects at risk of criminal or civil liability or be damaging to the subjects' financial standing, employability, or reputation.

3. Research involving the collection or study of existing data, documents, records, pathologic specimens, or diagnostic specimens, if these sources are publicly available or if the information is recorded by the investigator in such a manner that subjects cannot be identified, directly or through identifiers linked to the subjects.

Projects That May Be Reviewed by the IRB With an Expedited Procedure[1]

Expedited review can be carried out by the IRB chairperson or by one or more experienced reviewers. In reviewing the research, the reviewers may exercise all of the authorities of the IRB except that the reviewers may not disapprove the research. If the reviewers want to disprove the research, the review needs to go to the full committee. The expedited review process involves the same criteria as full-committee review, and there must be continuing review at least on an annual basis.

To approve a project with an expedited review process, the project must involve *no more than minimal risk*, and fit into one of these categories:

1. Clinical studies of drugs and medical devices only if an investigational new drug application is not required or an investigational device exemption application is not required; or the medical device is cleared/approved for marketing and the medical device is being used in accordance with its cleared/approved labeling.

---

[1]An expedited review procedure consists of a review of research involving human subjects by the IRB chairperson or by one or more experienced reviewers designated by the chairperson from among members of the IRB in accordance with the requirements set forth in 45 CFR 46.110.

2. Collection of blood samples by finger stick, heel stick, ear stick, or venipuncture as follows:
    a. from healthy, nonpregnant adults who weigh at least 110 pounds. For these subjects, the amounts drawn may not exceed 550 ml in an 8-week period, and collection may not occur more frequently than 2 times per week; or
    b. from other adults and children,[2] considering the age, weight, and health of the subjects, the collection procedure, the amount of blood to be collected, and the frequency with which it will be collected. For these subjects, the amount drawn may not exceed the lesser of 50 ml or 3 ml per kg in an 8-week period, and collection may not occur more frequently than 2 times per week.

3. Prospective collection of biologic specimens for research purposes by noninvasive means.

4. Collection of data through noninvasive procedures (not involving general anesthesia or sedation) routinely employed in clinical practice, excluding procedures involving X-rays or microwaves. Where medical devices are employed, they must be cleared/approved for marketing.

5. Research involving materials (data, documents, records, or specimens) that have been collected or will be collected solely for nonresearch purposes (such as medical treatment or diagnoses).

---

[2]Children are defined in the HHS regulations as "persons who have not attained the legal age for consent to treatments or procedures involved in the research, under the applicable law of the jurisdiction in which the research will be conducted." 45 CFR 46.402(a).

PART 2

THE FULL-COMMITTEE IRB MEETING

The Work Before an IRB Meeting

ROBERT AMDUR AND ELIZABETH A. BANKERT

Do the Work of IRB Review Before the Meeting

- Review your assigned information at least 2 days before the meeting.
- Consider the IRB meeting to be a place to discuss the issues and make decisions, not to gather information.
- Get your questions answered before the IRB meeting.
- Discuss your assignments with the investigator, other IRB members, or consultants prior to the IRB meeting.
- Do not hesitate to discuss the protocol with the investigator to facilitate the review process and promote mutual respect between the investigator and the IRB.
- Before the meeting, inform the IRB chairperson and/or other members if you have concerns about a proposal.
- Decide if the investigator should attend the meeting.
- If you want the investigator to make specific changes in the language of the application or consent document, then come to the meeting with the application rewritten so that it reads the way that you want it to read.

The purpose of this chapter is to emphasize the importance of doing the majority of the work of IRB review before the full-committee IRB meeting. Identifying and evaluating ethical issues are often time-consuming and complex processes. To be an effective IRB member, you have to be willing and able to conduct a thorough review of research proposals prior to the IRB meeting. The guidelines presented in this chapter apply to all types of agenda items—initial protocol review, revisions, and continuing reviews. For IRBs that use a primary reviewer system, these guidelines apply most directly to the IRB members who are assigned to a specific agenda item. The bottom line is, if you want to have a major impact on the protection of research subjects, then you have to follow the golden rule of IRB review: Do most of the work of IRB review *before* the meeting.

The guidelines listed in this chapter are specific behaviors that follow directly from the golden rule of IRB review.

• Review your assigned information at least 2 days before the meeting.

The IRB will not function optimally if members wait until the night before the meeting to review their assignments. Ideally, all IRB members will receive the paperwork they need at least 1 week before the meeting. At an absolute minimum, members should have 2 full days to work on their assignments.

• Consider the IRB meeting to be primarily a place to discuss the issues and make decisions, not to gather information.

An effective IRB will use the full-committee meeting time to debate issues and to make the difficult determinations that are required to meaningfully influence the protection of research subjects. It is counterproductive to use the meeting time for things that could have been done more effectively before the meeting.

- Get your questions answered *before* the IRB meeting.

A thorough IRB review usually means that you will need clarification or additional information about aspects of a research proposal. The IRB meeting is not the best place for most of these activities. Ideally, the IRB chairperson will establish clear expectations for each IRB member. Review your assignments ahead of time and come to the meeting with the information you need to make an informed recommendation about how the committee should vote on the issue.

- Discuss your assignments with the investigator, other IRB members, or consultants prior to the IRB meeting.

This is especially true for new protocol reviews but also applies to other types of assignments when the information presented is complex or troublesome. IRB members are not expected to be experts in the proposals that they review. Even when IRB members are knowledgeable about the type of research that they are reviewing, interaction with other people will be required to make informed determinations.

- Do not hesitate to discuss the protocol with the investigator.

Collegial interaction between investigators and IRB reviewers will facilitate the IRB review process and promote respect for the local IRB system. The IRB chairperson or administrative director should encourage members to directly contact investigators for further information or clarification. However, the IRB office should serve as an intermediary for any IRB member who wishes to obtain further information but does not have time to (or prefers not to) personally follow up with the investigator. Investigators who resist talking with IRB reviewers or who criticize them for requesting clarification or justification of important ethical issues demonstrate a lack of respect for the system of protecting research subjects that has been mandated by the organization for which the IRB serves.

- Before the meeting, inform the IRB chairperson and/or other IRB members if you have concerns about a proposal.

IRB reviewers should make every attempt to resolve issues and concerns prior to the meeting. This is not to suggest that there will not be issues that need to be discussed or debated at the full-committee meeting. An IRB that does not routinely struggle with controversial or potentially troublesome issues is probably not doing a good job.

When IRB members have issues that they are not able to resolve prior to a meeting, they should be sure that the IRB chairperson and other assigned reviewers are informed about the issues that concern them. This gives IRB members the opportunity to prepare for a knowledgeable discussion at the meeting.

- Decide whether or not the investigator should attend the meeting.

Some IRBs require an investigator to attend the IRB meeting with every new protocol review. Many IRBs find that it is not productive to require the investigator to attend the IRB meeting on a regular basis. When there is a question about whether the principal investigator or other important members of the research team will be present at the IRB meeting, it is important for the primary reviewers to decide if the investigator's presence at the meeting will facilitate IRB review of the protocol. When reviewers think that it will be useful for an investigator to attend the meeting, they should ask the IRB administrator to inform the investigator of this with as much lead time as possible.

The most common reason that the IRB would ask an investigator to attend the IRB meeting is to discuss an important issue that could not be resolved before the meeting. Another good reason might involve a situation where the reviewer thinks it will be important for other IRB members to hear an investigator explain something personally rather than to have the reviewer explain to the committee that there is no reason for concern. When an investigator is asked to attend the IRB meeting, the primary reviewer should explain to the investigator why his or her presence at the meeting may be useful.

- If you want the investigator to make specific changes in the language of the application or consent document, then come to the meeting with the application rewritten so that it reads the way that you want it to read.

IRB meeting time should be used to focus on complex or controversial issues. Respect for the IRB process is compromised when an IRB tables a proposal because the committee wants the investigator to change the way he or she answered a certain question on the IRB submission form or worded the research protocol. The consent process and document is the subject of a separate chapter. The IRB meeting is not the place to spend time polishing the wording of the consent document. In most cases, wording or response changes should be resolved with the investigator before the meeting. In cases where it is not possible to have the necessary revisions made prior to the meeting, the IRB reviewers should come to the meeting with an explicit recommendation for how the investigator should revise the proposal.

Reviewing a New Research Proposal

ROBERT AMDUR, SUSAN KORNETSKY,
AND SARAH KHAN

**Using a Systematic Approach to
Review a New Protocol Application**

- Establish a routine for reviewing the application package:
  1. Read the consent document, but do not take notes or make revisions.
  2. Read the protocol summary.
  3. Read the full protocol and supporting material carefully. Take notes as needed.
  4. Reread the consent document.
- Use a reviewer template, such as the one shown in this chapter.

Scenario: You have been assigned to be a primary reviewer for a new protocol and have just sat down to review the IRB application package a few days before the full-committee meeting. You are looking at a thick stack of papers that include things like an application checklist, a summary of the protocol, a detailed description of protocol procedures, and a consent document. You have to decide what to read first and how to structure your review. The purpose of this chapter is to suggest an approach that will make the process of your review more effective and more efficient.

Using a Systematic Approach to Review the Application Material

It is important to develop a formal system for reviewing the application material. What works well for one reviewer may not be the best system for another. Use the approach that works best for you. Some experienced IRB reviewers favor the following:

1. **Read the consent document.** Because the purpose of the consent document is to explain the important aspects of the study to potential subjects in lay language, it should give you a good introduction to the protocol. During this initial reading, you should not take notes or attempt to correct the wording of the document. The purpose of this reading is to orient you with the overall design of the study.

2. **Read the protocol summary.** After completing an overview of the study based on the consent form, review the summary of the protocol submitted as part of the IRB application. The IRB summary protocol is the part of the application where the investigator summarizes the important aspects of the study in a way that facilitates IRB review.

3. **Read the full protocol and supporting material.** Read the supporting material that completes the information presented in the IRB application form. For example, primary reviewers receive the full sponsor protocol from the study sponsor. This will provide the reviewer with detailed information such as prior studies that are applicable to the study treatment or that validate study procedures, statistical power analysis, detailed inclusion/exclusion requirements, and recruitment advertisements.

4. **Read the consent document again**. This time, record suggested corrections or questions for the investigator.

USING A REVIEWER TEMPLATE

A reviewer template is a form that lists the main issues or questions that an IRB reviewer evaluates when reviewing a new protocol. Such a template will help you to organize the review and to remember what issues have and have not been addressed. It is also useful for presenting the review at the full-committee meeting, and it can be kept in the IRB file as documentation that a detailed review was performed. Many reviewers create their own templates according to the format that works best for them, but some IRB offices ask every reviewer to use the same template, which in certain cases may be lengthy and extremely detailed. In our opinion, the primary purpose of the reviewer template is to help the reviewer evaluate the protocol and explain it to other IRB members. For this reason, it is useful to keep the template as short and simple as possible. A sample one-page template is included next. The most applicable Belmont Report principle is shown in boldface after each item to remind the reviewer why the information is important.

IRB Primary Reviewer Template

Study No.: _____
(Write on the other side of this page as needed.)
Reviewer: _____ Date: _____
Purpose of study:

Summary (background, number of arms, controls, IND, etc.):

Sponsor:

Investigator (Is he or she qualified? Does he or she have a conflict of interest?) **[Beneficence]**

continues

IRB Primary Reviewer Template
continued

<u>Study population and recruitment practices</u>
Includes vulnerable subjects (children, etc.)?
[Respect for persons]
Subject recruitment (who, where, how?) **[Beneficence]**
Payment or reimbursements (coercive?) **[Beneficence]**
Is subject selection likely to be equitable? **[Justice]**
Adequacy of procedures to protect vulnerable subjects
[Respect for persons]

<u>Informed consent (written, surrogate, etc.)</u>
[Respect for persons]

<u>Birth control</u> **[Beneficence]**

<u>Genetic testing/tissue repository</u>
[Respect for persons and beneficence]
Will the subjects or their doctors be given research results?
Are they informed of this before enrolling?

<u>Cost (relative to nonresearch cost)</u>
Will subjects understand increased cost? **[Respect for persons]**
Are subjects coerced to accept increased cost? **[Beneficence]**

<u>Risks (relative to nonresearch alternative)</u> **[Beneficence]**
Rate risk level as (1) minimal, (2) moderate, or (3) high:
Absolute _____ Relative _____
Risks are minimized. (Appropriate control group?)

<u>Potential benefit (direct for the subject versus altruism)</u>

<u>Risk/benefit analysis</u> **[Beneficence]**
Risks are minimized and reasonable in view of potential
benefits.

<u>Confidentiality</u> **[Respect for persons]**
Provisions to protect privacy and confidentiality are adequate.

<u>Data oversight</u> **[Beneficence]**
How will data be monitored?
Stopping rules are explained and sufficiently detailed.

<u>Consent document</u> **[Respect for persons]**
Accurately describes the essential elements in a way that is
likely to be understood by the expected subject population.

A MORE DETAILED REVIEWER WORKSHEET

A reviewer worksheet is a tool that assists IRB members in reviewing research protocols. In some institutions, the use of a worksheet is suggested; in others, the use of a worksheet is mandatory. This section presents a version of the worksheet that is used at Children's Hospital in Boston, Massachusetts.

The worksheet is divided into 12 sections; each addresses one of the criteria for IRB approval as specified in the regulations and presents specific questions and criteria to be considered. In addition, in some sections, members can write questions or concerns that an investigator needs to address. The worksheet sections thus prompt IRB members to make specific determinations for an individual protocol.

Reviewer Worksheet

INTRODUCTION, SPECIFIC AIMS, AND BACKGROUND

- Are the specific aims clearly specified?
- Are there adequate preliminary data to justify the research?
- Is there appropriate justification for this research protocol?

SCIENTIFIC DESIGN

- Is the scientific design adequate to answer the question?
- Are the objectives likely to be achievable within a given time period?
- Is the scientific design (i.e., randomization; placebo controls; Phase 1, 2, or 3) described and adequately justified?

INCLUSION/EXCLUSION CRITERIA FOR SUBJECTS

- Are inclusion and exclusion criteria clearly specified and appropriate?
- If women, minorities, or children are included or excluded, is this justified?

continues

Reviewer Worksheet *continued*

- Is the choice of subjects appropriate for the question being asked?
- Is the principle of distributive justice adequately incorporated into the inclusion and exclusion criteria for the research protocol? Is subject selection equitable?

RECRUITMENT OF SUBJECTS

- Are the methods for recruiting potential subjects well defined?
- Are the location and timing of the recruitment process acceptable?
- Is the individual performing the recruitment appropriate for the process?
- Are all recruitment materials submitted and appropriate?
- Are there acceptable methods for screening subjects before recruitment?

RESEARCH PROCEDURES

- Are the rationale and details of the research procedures accurately described and acceptable?
- Is there a clear differentiation between research procedures and standard care?
- Are the individuals performing the procedures appropriately educated?
- Is the location of where the procedure will be performed acceptable?
- Are there adequate plans to inform subjects about specific research results if necessary (clinically relevant results, risk of depression, risk of suicide, incidental findings, etc.)?

DRUGS, BIOLOGICS, AND DEVICES

- Is the status of the drug described and appropriate (investigational, new use of an FDA-approved drug, or an FDA-approved drug within approved indications)?
- Are the drug dosage and route of administration appropriate?
- Are the drug or device safety and efficacy data sufficient to warrant the proposed phase of testing?
- Is the significant risk or nonsignificant risk status of the device described and appropriate?

DATA ANALYSIS AND STATISTICAL ANALYSIS

- Is the rationale for the proposed number of subjects reasonable?
- Are the plans for data and statistical analysis defined and justified, including the use of stopping rules and end points?
- Are there adequate provisions for monitoring data, e.g., a data safety monitoring board (DSMB)?

POTENTIAL RISKS, DISCOMFORTS, AND BENEFITS FOR SUBJECTS

- Are the risks and benefits adequately identified, evaluated, and described?
- Are the potential risks minimized and the likelihood of benefits maximized?
- Is the risk/benefit ratio acceptable for proceeding with the research?
- If children are involved, which regulatory category of risk/benefit does the protocol fall within, and are all criteria within the category adequately addressed?

COMPENSATION AND COSTS FOR SUBJECTS

- Is the amount or type of compensation or reimbursement reasonable?
- Are there adequate provisions to avoid out-of-pocket expenses by the research subject, or is there sufficient justification to allow subjects to pay?
- If children or adolescents are involved, who receives the compensation, and is this appropriate?

PRIVACY AND CONFIDENTIALITY

- Are there adequate provisions to protect the privacy and ensure the confidentiality of the research subjects?
- Are there adequate plans to store and code the data?
- Is the use of identifiers or links to identifiers necessary, and how is this information protected?

INFORMED CONSENT/ASSENT

- Are all the elements of informed consent contained in the consent document?
- Is the process of obtaining consent adequately described?
- Is assent required?
- Is waiver or modification of consent possible?

continues

Reviewer Worksheet *continued*

OTHER ISSUES

- Are adequate references provided?
- When should the next review occur? If frequent reviews are necessary, how should the interval be determined?

The Consent Process and Document

ROBERT AMDUR AND ELIZABETH A. BANKERT

INFORMATION THAT MUST BE PROVIDED TO POTENTIAL SUBJECTS

- Research purpose and procedures
- Risks and discomforts
- Potential benefits
- Alternative procedures or treatments
- Provisions for confidentiality
- Management of research-related injury
- Contacts for additional information
- Voluntary participation and the right to discontinue participation without penalty

INFORMATION THAT MUST BE PROVIDED WHEN APPLICABLE

- Unforeseeable risks
- Termination of participation by the investigator
- Additional costs
- Consequences of discontinuing research participation
- Notification of significant new findings
- Approximate number of subjects

It is the responsibility of the investigator to obtain informed consent from potential subjects. The research community depends on the integrity of the investigator to successfully complete the consent process. Investigators should acknowledge that in some cases, obtaining informed consent will be a difficult task.

A role of the IRB is to ensure the investigator provides appropriate information to potential subjects. This information is most often depicted in a consent document. However, the *process* of obtaining consent merits as much attention from the investigator and IRB. Both the consent *process* and *document* are important.

The consent process should take place in an environment free from coercion and without undue influence. Components of consent include voluntariness, disclosure of relevant information, and determination of comprehension. The dialog between subject and investigator should continue throughout the study. Tools have been developed to enhance this dialog. One such tool we created is referred to as the informed consent evaluation feedback tool (ICE FT). This tool provides questions to the potential subject in advance of and during the consent process. This type of instrument should aid in improving comprehension of subjects by increasing dialog.

It is important for the consent document to be written clearly and concisely. Please note, however, the use of committee time to revise the consent document is not efficient. Committee time should not be focused on wordsmithing. Rather, the primary reviewers should take time prior to the meeting to ensure the consent document is clear.

There are efforts throughout the research community to evaluate and improve the format of the consent document in an attempt to increase research subject comprehension. One concept is to include a summary of the research study at the beginning of the consent document to provide a brief, clear overview of the study. IRB administrators should maintain an awareness of these efforts and apprise IRB members of best practices.

IRBs need to understand the wide variety of types of research and should be able to work with investigators to ensure both the process and the document are optimal. Investigators should describe the consent process within the application to the IRB and state whether or not there are other members of the research team to whom the investigator has delegated this responsibility.

Here are some guidelines that IRB members should follow when reviewing the consent document:

- Use the term *consent document* or *consent form* instead of *informed consent*. Informed consent indicates an action—an ongoing process of communication between the subject and research staff—is occurring. Informed consent is not a document, and presenting subjects with information in a document does not constitute informed consent on their part.
- Resist the urge to make unimportant changes to the consent document. Every consent form can be improved with slightly different wording. It is important to ensure that the consent form clearly describes the elements discussed later in this chapter; however, polishing and wordsmithing the document will not meaningfully improve the protection of research subjects. When considering a change in the consent document, ask yourself, "Is this change likely to have an important impact on the protection of research subjects?" If the answer is "no," then do not make the change.
- If you want to revise the consent document, then record your changes in writing before the IRB meeting. Minor changes can be submitted directly to the IRB staff and need not be described during the IRB meeting.
- If you want to make substantive changes, such as adding major risks or eliminating potential benefits, then make an effort to discuss the changes with the investigator before the meeting. It is important to identify issues of contention before the meeting so that all parties can explain their view before the IRB makes a determination.
- The consent document should be written in lay language. Although it is difficult to define what is meant by *lay language*, the consent document should be written so that the intended subject population is likely to

understand the important information. There is much talk about requiring the consent document to be written at the eighth-grade level, and there are word processing programs that profess to evaluate this. Most IRBs find these programs of little value because the concepts are artificial. There is no substitute for having someone read the consent document and make subjective decisions about the complexity of the language.

• The primary reviewer should determine that the consent process and document contains information required by federal regulations. Federal regulations list 8 essential elements of informed consent and require that additional information be explained in certain circumstances. Because the first required element has 4 subsections, there are actually 14 items that the consent document should contain.

INFORMATION THAT MUST BE PROVIDED TO POTENTIAL SUBJECTS

1. **Research purpose and procedures**: A statement that the study involves research, an explanation of the purposes of the research, the expected duration of the subject's participation, a description of the procedures to be followed, and identification of any procedures that are experimental.

2. **Risks and discomforts**: A description of any reasonably foreseeable risks or discomforts to the subject.

3. **Potential benefits**: A description of any benefits to the subject or to others that may reasonably be expected from the research.

4. **Alternative procedures or treatments**: A disclosure of appropriate alternative procedures or courses of treatment, if any, that might be advantageous to the subject.

5. **Provisions for confidentiality**: A statement describing the extent, if any, to which confidentiality of records identifying the subject will be maintained.

6. **Management of research-related injury**: For research involving more than minimal risk, an explanation as to whether any compensation and any medical treatments are available if injury occurs and, if so, what they consist of, or where further information may be obtained.

7. **Contacts for additional information**: An explanation of whom to contact for answers to pertinent questions about the research and research subject's rights, and whom to contact in the event of a research-related injury to the subject.

8. **Voluntary participation and the right to discontinue participation without penalty**: A statement that participation is voluntary; refusal to participate will involve no penalty or loss of benefits to which the subject is otherwise entitled, and the subject may discontinue participation at any time without penalty or loss of benefits to which the subject is otherwise entitled.

When appropriate, the following information must be provided:

9. **Unforeseeable risks**: A statement that the particular treatment or procedure may involve risks to the subject (or to the embryo or fetus, if the subject is or may become pregnant) that are currently unforeseeable.

10. **Termination of participation by the investigator**: Anticipated circumstances under which the subject's participation may be terminated by the investigator without regard to the subject's consent.

11. **Additional costs**: Any additional costs to the subject that may result from participation in the research.

12. **Consequences of discontinuing research participation**: The consequences of a subject's decision to withdraw from the research and procedures for orderly termination of participation by the subject.

13. **Notification of significant new findings**: A statement that significant new findings developed during the course of the research that may relate to the subject's willingness to continue participation will be provided to the subject.

14. **Approximate number of subjects**: The approximate number of subjects involved in the study.

Continuing
Review of
Research

ROBERT AMDUR

Guidelines for Continuing Review of Research

- Determine if the study is currently enrolling, treating, or following subjects.
- Determine that the number of subjects enrolled at the IRB's institution does not exceed the initially approved number.
- Review any requested protocol revisions and any protocol revisions that have been approved by the IRB since the last continuing review.
- Determine if the study is progressing as planned.
- Determine if unexpected events have occurred that may indicate a need for a change in the protocol or consent document.
- Determine if information has become available since starting the study that indicates a need for modifications.
- Determine if subjects have registered any grievances or complaints about this study.
- Determine whether the consent document that is currently in use contains all previously approved revisions.
- Review a current report from the data monitoring mechanism to determine that study events are being evaluated relative to the appropriate stopping or modification rules.

In 2007, the OHRP updated guidance information about continuing review of research by the IRB. The text in this chapter is taken directly from the 2007 OHRP guidance document.

WHAT CONSTITUTES SUBSTANTIVE AND MEANINGFUL CONTINUING REVIEW?

Continuing review of research must be substantive and meaningful. Federal guidelines describe the criteria that must be satisfied in order for the IRB to approve research. These criteria include, among other things, determinations by the IRB regarding risks, potential benefits, informed consent, and safeguards for human subjects. The IRB must ensure that these criteria are satisfied at the time of both initial and continuing review. In particular, when conducting continuing review, the IRB needs to determine whether any new information has emerged—either from the research itself or from other sources—that could alter the IRB's previous determinations, particularly with respect to risk to subjects. Of note, information regarding any unanticipated problems involving risks to subjects or others (hereinafter referred to as unanticipated problems) that have occurred since the previous IRB review in most cases will be pertinent to the IRB's determinations at the time of continuing review.

In conducting continuing review of research not eligible for expedited review, all IRB members should at least receive and review a protocol summary and a status report on the progress of the research that includes:

- the number of subjects accrued;
- a summary of any unanticipated problems and available information regarding adverse events (in many cases, such a summary could be a simple brief statement that there have been no unanticipated problems and that adverse events have occurred at the expected frequency and level of severity as documented in the

research protocol, the informed consent document, and any investigator brochure);
- a summary of any withdrawal of subjects from the research since the last IRB review;
- a summary of any complaints about the research since the last IRB review;
- a summary of any recent literature that may be relevant to the research and any amendments or modifications to the research since the last IRB review;
- any relevant multi-center trial reports;
- any other relevant information, especially information about risks associated with the research; and
- a copy of the current informed consent document and any newly proposed consent document.

At least one member of the IRB (i.e., a primary reviewer) also should receive a copy of the complete protocol including any modifications previously approved by the IRB. Furthermore, upon request, any IRB member also should have access to the complete IRB protocol file and relevant IRB minutes prior to or during the convened IRB meeting.

When reviewing the current informed consent document(s), the IRB should ensure the following:

- The currently approved or proposed consent document is still accurate and complete;
- Any significant new findings that may relate to the subject's willingness to continue participation are provided to the subject in accordance with HHS regulations at 45 CFR 46.116(b)(5).

Review of currently approved or newly proposed consent documents must occur during the scheduled continuing review of research by the IRB, but informed consent documents should be reviewed whenever new information becomes available that would require modification of information in the informed consent document.

WHAT ARE SOME ADDITIONAL CONSIDERATIONS FOR CONTINUING REVIEW OF MULTICENTER TRIALS MONITORED BY A DSMB, DMC, OTHER SIMILAR BODY, OR SPONSOR?

As noted previously, continuing review of research by the IRB should include consideration of, among other things, unanticipated problems, adverse events, and any recent literature that may be relevant to the research.

OHRP recognizes that local investigators participating in multicenter clinical trials usually are unable to prepare a meaningful summary of adverse events for their IRBs because study-wide information regarding adverse events is not readily available to them. In such circumstances, when the clinical trial is subject to oversight by a monitoring entity (e.g., the research sponsor, a coordinating or statistical center, or a DSMB/data monitoring committee [DMC]), OHRP recommends that at the time of continuing review local investigators submit to their IRBs a current report from the monitoring entity. OHRP further recommends that such reports include the following:

(1) a statement indicating what information (e.g., study-wide adverse events, interim findings, and any recent literature that may be relevant to the research) was reviewed by the monitoring entity;

(2) the date of the review; and

(3) the monitoring entity's assessment of the information reviewed.

It may also be appropriate for the IRB at the time of continuing review to confirm that any provisions under the previously approved protocol for monitoring study data to ensure safety of subjects have been implemented and are working as intended (e.g., the IRB could require that the investigator provide a report from the monitoring entity described in the IRB-approved protocol).

REFERENCE

Office for Human Research Protections. (2007). *Guidance on continuing review.* Available: http://www.hhs.gov/ohrp/humansubjects/guidance/contrev0107.htm.

Protocol Revisions

ROBERT AMDUR

Guidelines for Review of Protocol Revisions

1. Identify the general category of information being revised:
   - Administrative details
   - Inclusion or exclusion criteria
   - Testing frequency or methods
   - Treatment parameters
   - Stopping or modification rules
   - Consent document
   - Recruitment procedures

2. Determine if the revision increases risk for currently enrolled subjects.

3. Determine if the revision increases risk for *future* subjects.

4. Determine if the consent document should be revised or if the proposed revision to the consent document is adequate.

5. Determine if consent should be obtained again from currently enrolled subjects.

6. If the proposed revision increases risk to current or future subjects, then determine if the protocol still meets the criteria that are used to evaluate new studies.

Federal regulations require that the IRB approve all research study revisions prior to their implementation. Regulations permit IRBs to review minimal risk revisions with an expedited process. Revisions that increase the risk of research participation or are more than a minor change to the protocol must be approved by the full IRB committee. It is for this reason that IRB members will be assigned to review protocol revisions as separate agenda items at the full-committee meeting.

The criteria for approving a protocol revision are the same as for approval of a new research proposal. Similarly, any proposed revision to the consent document must meet the requirements for initial approval of a consent document. Most IRBs use a separate form to guide the review of proposed revisions. Here are the main questions that an IRB member should focus on when reviewing a protocol revision:

1. What is the general category of information that is being revised?
   - Administrative details (research personnel, phone numbers, etc.)
   - Inclusion or exclusion criteria
   - Testing frequency or methods (a new questionnaire, more frequent blood draws, etc.)
   - Treatment parameters
   - Stopping or modification rules
   - Consent document
   - Recruitment procedures (payment schedules, advertisements, etc.)

2. Does the revision increase risk for currently enrolled subjects? Answers may include one of the following:
   - The revision does not increase risk.
   - The risk of the revision is minimal.
   - The risk of the revision is more than minimal.

3. Does the revision increase risk for future subjects? Answers may include one of the following:
   - The revision does not increase risk.
   - The risk of the revision is minimal.
   - The risk of the revision is more than minimal.

4. If the revision is not to the consent document, then should the consent document be revised as well?

5. Should consent be obtained again from currently enrolled subjects, and, if so, are there provisions to do so?

6. If the proposed revision increases risk to current or future subjects, then does the protocol still meet the criteria that are used to approve a new study?

Data and Safety Monitoring and Adverse Event Reporting

ROBERT AMDUR AND ELIZABETH A. BANKERT

IRB Review of Adverse Event Reports

- The role of the IRB is to ensure the research plan makes adequate provisions for monitoring the data collected to ensure the safety of subjects.
- Events reported to the IRB should be unanticipated; possibly related; and place subjects at a greater risk of harm than was previously known.
- Evaluate risk/benefit profile of research participation and whether or not a comparison of the observed and expected frequency of the event in the study population should be made.
- Should the protocol or consent document be revised?
- Should currently enrolled subjects be reconsented?
- Should the frequency or nature of continuing IRB review be changed to monitor the study more closely as a result of the adverse event?

There are federal regulations describing reporting requirements of adverse events for the investigator, the sponsor, the FDA, and the IRB. The reporting requirements for these entities are not the same. In addition, the reporting requirements are not the same for drugs as for medical devices.

An important role of the IRB is to ensure, when appropriate, the research plan makes adequate provision for monitoring the data collected to ensure the safety of subjects. This regulatory criterion does *not* state the IRB must serve as a data safety monitoring board. Previous to 2007, IRBs were inundated with adverse event forms. Fortunately, however, OHRP updated guidance related to adverse event reporting in a document entitled, *Guidance on Reviewing and Reporting Unanticipated Problems Involving Risks to Subjects or Others and Adverse Events*. The FDA has also recently released guidance on this topic. These guidance documents contain important information and should be carefully reviewed.

The OHRP guidance document describes the following elements, which may be included in an adequate data safety monitoring plan: type of data or events that are to be captured; entity responsible for monitoring the data collected, including data related to unanticipated problems and adverse events, and their respective roles (e.g., the investigators, the research sponsor, a coordinating or statistical center, an independent medical monitor, a DSMB/DMC, and/or some other entity); time frames for reporting adverse events and unanticipated problems to the monitoring entity; frequency of assessments of data or events captured by the monitoring provisions; definition of specific triggers or stopping rules that will dictate when some action is required; as appropriate, procedures for communicating to the IRB(s), the study sponsor, the investigator(s), and other appropriate officials the outcome of the reviews by the monitoring entity.

Once the IRB has approved the data and safety monitoring plan, the IRB office should use forms to collect appropriate information and to assist the IRB review processes related to adverse event reporting. Two forms should capture the information needed for IRB review: (1) Reporting Form for an Unanticipated Problem Involving Risks to Subjects or Others and (2) Serious Adverse Event and Unanticipated Adverse Device Effect Reporting Form for Clinical Trials.

Information collected should include:

- Confirmation that the events being reported should be unanticipated; possibly related to the research; and that the research places subjects or others at a greater risk of harm than was previously known or recognized.
- A description of the event.
- Location of event (on site or off site); determination if report is a follow-up to a previously reported event.
- Determination as to whether or not the event required action to protect other subjects. If yes, a description of the action and its urgency should be included.
- Determination as to whether or not the consent document or any part of the study plan should be revised as a result of the event. If yes, a description should be included.
- Determination as to whether or not currently enrolled subjects will be notified of the incident. If yes, a description of the notification process should be included.

In the Serious Adverse Event and Unanticipated Adverse Device Effect Reporting Form for Clinical Trials, additional items should be reviewed, including seriousness and detailed information related to the event, such as whether or not the information is contained in the investigator's brochure. A more detailed discussion of items to ask the researcher and the IRB review of responses follows.

In view of the confusion about the guidelines for adverse event reporting, it is not unusual to see events come before the IRB that were anticipated in this study population. Although it is our opinion that such events need not be reviewed by the IRB because they are not unanticipated, some duplication in the review form is useful to clarify the important issues. An event that is described in the consent document or protocol summary was clearly anticipated prior to starting the study. The event may be unanticipated in frequency, but it is not unexpected to observe the event in some of the study subjects.

Another reason to determine if the adverse event is currently described in the consent document is that IRB review of an adverse event report should include a decision about revising the consent document and reobtaining consent from enrolled subjects.

The local-versus-outside distinction is important in multisite studies. A local adverse event is an event that occurred in an institution for which the relevant IRB is directly responsible. An outside event is one that occurred at an institution for which the IRB is not responsible.

We include this question because many discussions of this subject in the literature make an important distinction between those events that are, versus those that are not, related to research participation. Although this certainly is an important issue, the point of adverse event monitoring is to review events that could change the risk of research participation. Therefore, from the standpoint of research regulation or research ethics, the term *adverse event* refers only to events that are or could be caused by research participation. Events that are clearly not related to research participation should not be reported to the IRB or discussed in the context of research regulation because they have no impact on the ethics of research conduct.

OBSERVED VERSUS EXPECTED FREQUENCY COMPARISON

- Does a determination of the implication of this adverse event for the risk/benefit profile of research participation require a comparison of the observed and expected frequency of this event in the study population?

If your answer to this question is "yes," then answer the next question.

- Is the observed-to-expected comparison being evaluated at the appropriate intervals by a person or group that is qualified to make the comparisons in a time frame that will protect the welfare of research participants?

If your answer to this question is "yes," then answer the next question.

- Who is making the comparisons required to appropriately evaluate this adverse event? Principal investigator _____; data monitoring committee _____; independent data safety monitoring board _____

The concept that many events can only be interpreted by calculating observed and expected frequency rates is difficult for some people to understand, and many IRBs and investigators are not used to thinking in these terms. However, it is essential that IRB members understand the limitations of IRB review of individual adverse event reports. In most settings, the main risk of research participation is not that a totally unknown toxicity will occur, but rather that an expected toxicity or adverse outcome will occur at a higher than expected frequency.

For example, consider a trial that involves a randomized comparison of best standard therapy plus or minus an investigational drug designed to improve survival following a heart attack. A major risk of study participation is that the study drug will do something harmful that leads to decreased survival. However, most IRBs have no way to evaluate the issue of increased mortality from individual adverse event reports. The IRB will usually not have the denominator needed to make frequency calculations, the resources available to perform the necessary statistical comparisons, or the expertise available to make observed versus expected comparisons in a given study population. There is no way for the IRB to get this information, and the IRB should not attempt to do so.

Federal regulations require the IRB to determine that the research plan provides for the monitoring of data in a way that will protect the welfare of research participants, but multiple federal guidance documents clearly explain that the IRB is not expected to be that mechanism with many types of studies. At the time of initial protocol review, the IRB is supposed to determine if the principal investigator, a data-monitoring committee, or an independent data safety monitoring board will monitor data in an ongoing manner from the standpoint of subject safety and that the details of the monitoring process are appropriate. In multicenter trials, or in any trial where the study populations are large, meaningful IRB review of an adverse event report requires that the IRB determine that someone other than the IRB is monitoring the event as planned.

CHANGE IN THE RISK/BENEFIT PROFILE

- Does this adverse event suggest that there is a meaningful change in the risk/benefit profile of research participation for subjects who are currently enrolled in the study?
- If this adverse event does suggest that the risk/benefit profile of research participation has changed, then should the study protocol (the methods, inclusion/exclusion criteria, etc.) be revised to minimize the risk of research participation (including the option of study suspension or closure)?

If this adverse event does suggest that the risk/benefit profile of research participation has changed, then a determination about the need to revise the study protocol and/or the consent document must be made. The IRB should review the responses of the investigator and then make its own determinations by considering the following questions:

- Is a revision in the study protocol required to minimize the risk of research participation?

- Should the document be revised to discuss the adverse event?
- Should the investigator reobtain consent from currently enrolled subjects?
- Should the frequency or nature of IRB continuing review of this protocol be changed to monitor the study more closely as a result of this adverse event?

The IRB administrator and IRB chairperson should review the forms and document the outcome of the initial review of the incident. Outcome may include one of the following: (1) no further action is required; (2) full committee review is required; (3) report to OHRP is required; or (4) further information is required to complete the review.

Primary Reviewer Presentations

ROBERT AMDUR AND ELIZABETH A. BANKERT

Guidelines for Primary Reviewer Presentations

- Limit the initial summary of your review to 1–2 minutes.
- Your presentation should consist of reading your review form.
- Resist the urge to impress the committee with how much work you did.
- Presentations by secondary reviewers should focus on areas of disagreement with previous reviewers.
- Do not allow questions until after all of the primary and secondary reviewers have made their presentations.
- End your presentation with a vote recommendation.

For an IRB to function optimally, it is important that IRB members use an organized format for presenting their reviews at a full-committee meeting. Each type of IRB review (new protocols, continuing review, protocol revisions, or adverse event reports) should have a specialized review form that helps the reviewer conduct and present his or her evaluation. The purpose of this chapter is to give IRB members guidelines about presenting their reviews to the rest of the committee.

- Limit the initial summary of your review to 1–2 minutes.

All IRB members should receive the main documents from all study applications prior to the full-committee meeting. The primary reviewer should begin with a brief summary of the project. The purpose of an initial presentation is to summarize the important points of the IRB review. The primary reviewers should complete their presentations before the discussion is opened to other committee members.

- Your presentation should consist of reading your review form.

If you use a good review form and organize the information in writing before the meeting, reading what you have recorded on your review form is the best way to present your review to other IRB members.

- Resist the urge to impress the committee with how much work you did.

A high-quality review often requires many hours of hard work on the part of a primary reviewer. The review may include discussions with the principal investigator and consultants, the reading of related literature, and clarification of initially confusing protocol information. There is a natural tendency for the primary reviewer to want to impress colleagues by making them relive the trials and tribulations of the review experience.

It is important for IRB members to recognize that the committee expects and appreciates a thorough review on the part of each primary reviewer but that optimal IRB function requires only a summary at the IRB meeting. This is not to say that IRB members should not explain the efforts that they went through to evaluate a protocol item or the complex issues that they encountered. It is both important and appropriate for primary reviewers to explain to the IRB committee and to document on a review form the important events in the review process, including significant time factors. However, it is possible to summarize this information in a way that gives the committee the facts needed to make an informed determination without making them relive a reviewer's experience.

• Presentations by secondary reviewers should focus on areas of disagreement with previous reviewers.

When there is more than one primary reviewer assigned to an agenda item, all successive reviewers should focus the presentation of their review on the areas where they disagree with the previous reviewer(s) or have additional comments. Subsequent reviewers should communicate their evaluations by also reviewing the list of important issues to consider and stating whether they agree or disagree with the information that was presented by previous reviewers. If there is disagreement or there are different interpretations, then this should be explained to the committee.

• Do not allow questions until after all of the primary and secondary reviewers have made their presentations.

In many situations, IRB members will want to ask questions to clarify their understanding of a primary reviewer's summary presentation. The IRB will function better if the IRB meeting is structured so that both the primary and secondary reviewers complete their summary presentations before discussing comments or questions from other IRB members.

• End your presentation with a vote recommendation.

There are many situations where a primary or secondary reviewer wants to consider the opinions of other IRB members before finalizing a decision on how to vote on an agenda item. This is how the IRB should function, and all IRB members should keep an open mind throughout full-committee discussions. However, it will improve the IRB review process if both primary and secondary reviewers approach their assignments with a goal of being able to end their initial presentation with a recommendation for how the committee should vote on the item in question. All IRB members should understand that such recommendations should be viewed as preliminary assessments that are being included in the initial presentations to help committee members clarify their thinking on the important issues.

All IRB members should be aware of the criteria for IRB approval of research per 45 CFR 46.111 (outlined in the following box).

Criteria for IRB Approval of Research per 45 CFR 46.111

In order to approve research, the IRB shall determine that all of the following requirements are satisfied:

- Risks to subjects are minimized by using procedures that are consistent with sound research design and that do not unnecessarily expose subjects to risk, and whenever appropriate, by using procedures already being performed on the subjects for diagnostic or treatment purposes.
- Risks to subjects are reasonable in relation to anticipated benefits, if any, to subjects, and the importance of the knowledge that may reasonably be expected to result. In evaluating risks and benefits, the IRB should consider only those risks and benefits that may result from the research (as distinguished from risks and benefits of therapies subjects would receive even if not participating in the research). The IRB should not consider possible long-range effects of applying knowledge gained in the research (for example, the possible effects of the research on public policy) as among those research risks that fall within the purview of its responsibility.
- Selection of subjects is equitable. In making this assessment, the IRB should take into account the purposes of the research and the setting in which the research will be conducted and should be particularly cognizant of the special problems of research

involving vulnerable populations, such as children, prisoners, pregnant women, mentally disabled persons, or economically or educationally disadvantaged persons.

- Informed consent will be sought from each prospective subject or the subject's legally authorized representative.
- Informed consent will be appropriately documented.
- When appropriate, the research plan makes adequate provision for monitoring the data collected to ensure the safety of subjects.
- When appropriate, there are adequate provisions to protect the privacy of subjects and to maintain the confidentiality of data.
- When some or all of the subjects are likely to be vulnerable to coercion or undue influence, such as children, prisoners, pregnant women, mentally disabled persons, or economically or educationally disadvantaged persons, additional safeguards have been included in the study to protect the rights and welfare of these subjects.

Deciding
How to Vote

ROBERT AMDUR AND ELIZABETH A. BANKERT

The Five Vote Options

1. Approved as submitted
2. Minor revisions required
3. Not approved (substantial revisions required)
4. Recuse
5. Abstain

Each member of the IRB lends his/her unique expertise to the group dynamic and to the decision-making process. As a whole, the IRB must include individuals with varying backgrounds and through this diversity allow for consideration of "race, gender, and cultural backgrounds and sensitivity to such issues as community attitudes" (45 CFR 46.107). Professional experience is required to review specific research activities and to "ascertain the acceptability of proposed research in terms of institutional commitments and regulations and standards of professional conduct and practice" (45 CFR 46.107). In addition, if an IRB regularly reviews research involving "children, prisoners, pregnant women, handicapped or mentally disabled persons, consideration should be given to the inclusion of knowledgeable individuals working with this subject population" (45 CFR 46.107).

We want to emphasize that although specific expertise is required, it is important to understand each IRB member should use the same standards in evaluating and voting on a proposed project. There is sometimes a misconception that the nonaffiliated or nonscientific member have a significantly different role relative to the other IRB members. Indeed, scientific members are expected to adequately describe the proposed project so that all IRB members understand the research. However, meeting discussions should center around core ethical principles as outlined in this handbook. Each IRB member should be comfortable in stating his or her issues and should not feel intimidated. The role of the IRB chairperson is extremely important in ensuring each member has ample opportunity to voice concerns and ask questions.

After the primary reviewers have presented their summaries and the full committee has discussed the agenda item, there comes a time when IRB members must each decide how they are going to vote. In some IRBs, the chairperson determines when the discussion is sufficient to call for a vote, while in others, a vote call requires the support of at least two IRB members. Suggested voting options:

- **Approved as submitted**: This means that the investigator is not required to change any aspect of the protocol or consent document. The approval is valid for 1 year unless the committee designates a shorter period due to the risk of the study.
- **Minor revisions required**: This means that the full committee does not need to review the study again unless the researcher fails to provide *simple concurrence* with the minor revisions that the IRB has requested. The letter to the investigator must tell the investigator exactly what revisions to make and that the study may not begin until the IRB chairperson (or designee) has approved the revisions and issued a final letter of approval.
- **Not approved (substantial revisions required)**: This means that the magnitude or number of concerns, questions, or problems is such that the full IRB committee must review a revised study application.
- **Recuse**: If an IRB member has a conflict of interest with any part of the study, the IRB member should

not participate in the initial or continuing review of the study except to provide information requested by the IRB. He or she must leave the room and not participate in the vote. This is considered a *recusal* and will not be counted as part of the voting quorum. Conflicts of interest include financial interest, active participation in the trial as principal investigator or co-principal investigator, or any other issue for which the member feels his or her vote could be considered potentially conflicted.

- **Abstain**: If an IRB member does not have a conflict but feels that he or she should not vote on a study, the member may *abstain* from voting. A vote to *abstain* will be included as part of the voting quorum. An abstention vote should be a rare event. The typical reason that an IRB member abstains from voting is when he or she was not present for discussion of an important issue. When an IRB member has been present for discussion of the major issues, but is still not comfortable approving the study item, then he or she should register a *not approved* vote.

There will be many situations where it is difficult for IRB members to decide how to vote. The most common scenario is that an IRB member is concerned about some aspect of the protocol but is not sure if voting to not approve the item is justified.

There is no way to eliminate the tension and uncertainty that is often associated with making IRB determinations. The nature of IRB work is that IRB members will frequently be required to make important decisions without definitive guidance. Two guidelines will help IRB members structure their thinking on how to vote at the IRB meeting:

1. **Use the three ethical principles described in the Belmont Report to analyze and explain concerns about research procedures**. The Belmont Report, discussed in Chapter 1-4, presents the principles of respect for persons, beneficence, and justice. These are the tools that IRB members should use to

analyze research procedures. It is much easier to evaluate important IRB issues and to explain concerns to other IRB members if one has a language for discussing the ethical standards of research involving human subjects. The Belmont Report gives IRB members the language they need to explain why they are concerned about a research procedure in a way that gets to the core ethical issues and is consistent from one discussion to another.

2. **Vote "No."**: IRB members should vote to not approve a protocol if there is doubt about an ethical principle or if there is not enough information presented to allow for a decision. The research protocol will be reviewed again by the full committee. It is important to clearly describe the issues to the investigator via the letter from the IRB.

IRB members should take the approach that the information reviewed by the IRB—including discussion at the IRB meeting—should provide all the information that they need to feel that it is acceptable to approve the protocol under discussion. IRB members should never be told that their concern about an issue is unwarranted because they don't understand the details of the situation. IRB members do not need to understand complex scientific information or procedures to evaluate core ethical issues. IRB members with expertise in the research under discussion should be able to explain the research in a way that allows all IRB members to understand the important information. If IRB members do not understand the information provided or feel that they cannot make an informed decision based on the information, they should vote to not approve the protocol until they arrive at the level of understanding needed to make an informed decision.

DETERMINATION OF RISK LEVEL

The determination of risk level is a requirement of research being conducted at Veterans Administration (VA) facilities.

Some non-VA IRBs have also implemented this determination. The IRB's decision is between minimal risk and greater than minimal risk and must be documented in the minutes. According to the regulations, the definition of minimal risk means that the probability and magnitude of harm or discomfort anticipated in the research are not greater in and of themselves than those ordinarily encountered in daily life or during the performance of routine physical or psychological examinations or tests. This discussion should focus on the *research* aspects of the protocol.

REFERENCE

Protection of Human Subjects, 45 C. F. R. pt. 46 (2009).

SPECIFIC TOPICS

Evaluating Study Design and Quality

ROBERT AMDUR

The IRB Must Evaluate Study Design and Scientific Quality

Ethical codes and federal regulations require that the IRB evaluate the study design and scientific quality. For example:

- Declaration of Helsinki (WMA, 2008): 12. Medical research involving human subjects must conform to generally accepted scientific principles and be based on a thorough knowledge of the scientific literature, other relevant sources of information, and adequate laboratory and, where appropriate, animal experimentation.
- Federal Regulation 45 CFR 46.111(a): Criteria for IRB approval of research: Risks to subjects are minimized by using procedures which are consistent with sound research design, and which do not, unnecessarily, expose subjects to risk.

It is not unusual for IRB members, institutional officials, and researchers to debate the role of the IRB in evaluating study design or factors that affect the quality of the science of research. For example, is it appropriate for IRB members to vote not to approve a study because they believe study results would be more persuasive if a different control group was used, or because previously completed research has already answered the study question? Is it appropriate for the IRB to question the validity of the statistical power calculation used to determine the number of subjects in a study? Some members of the research community are under the impression that it is not the role of the IRB to routinely evaluate the quality of the science of a protocol. Many IRB chairpersons have been confronted with statements like, "The IRB's job is to evaluate ethics. The IRB has no business commenting on the science of a study."

The purpose of this chapter is to explain the role of the IRB in evaluating study design and the other features of a study that may affect scientific quality. The bottom line is that there is no question that the IRB not only has the authority to evaluate scientific quality, but it also has the obligation to do so if it is to function in compliance with accepted ethical codes and federal research regulations.

ETHICS CODES

Nuremberg Code (1949)

Several sections of the Nuremberg Code address scientific quality and the risk/benefit profile. Point 3 is representative:

> The experiment should be so designed and based on the results of animal experimentation and knowledge of the natural history of the disease or other problem under study that the anticipated results will justify the performance of the experiment. (Nuremberg Code, 1947)

Declaration of Helsinki

Multiple sections of this ethical code address specific aspects of study design. It is a worthwhile document to read in total. In addition to item 12 cited above, other sections including 18, 21, and 32 are especially relevant to the question of IRB review of scientific quality:

> 18. Every medical research study involving human subjects must be preceded by careful assessment of pre-

dictable risks and burdens to the individuals and communities involved in the research in comparison with foreseeable benefits to them and to other individuals or communities affected by the condition under investigation.

21. Medical research involving human subjects may only be conducted if the importance of the objective outweighs the inherent risks and burdens to the research subjects.

32. The benefits, risks, burdens and effectiveness of a new intervention must be tested against those of the best current proven intervention, except in the following circumstances:
  • The use of placebo, or no treatment, is acceptable in studies where no current proven intervention exists; or
  • Where for compelling and scientifically sound methodological reasons the use of placebo is necessary to determine the efficacy or safety of an intervention and the patients who receive placebo or no treatment will not be subject to any risk of serious or irreversible harm. Extreme care must be taken to avoid abuse of this option.

(WMA, 2008)

FEDERAL RESEARCH REGULATIONS

HHS and corresponding FDA regulations require the IRB to determine that a study is designed so that risks to subjects are minimized and are justified by potential benefits. For example, these guidelines are offered in 45 CFR 46.111(a), Criteria for IRB approval of Research: "(1) Risks to subjects are minimized: (i) by using procedures which are consistent with sound research design, and which do not, unnecessarily, expose subjects to risk."

The IRB's Responsibility to Evaluate Scientific Quality

The IRB needs to act in compliance with federal research regulations and to make decisions that support the ethical principles in accepted ethical codes such as the Nuremberg Code and the Declaration of Helsinki. The sections from these guidance documents reproduced previously emphasize that a characteristic of ethical research is that (1) the study is designed so that the risks to subjects are minimized and (2) the potential benefits of the research justify the potential risks. It is these two directives that establish the obligation of the IRB to carefully consider the study design and overall scientific quality of each study.

The Study Design

If revising the study design will meaningfully decrease the risk to subjects without a major compromise in the persuasiveness of the study results, then the IRB should not approve the protocol. Similarly, when a study that involves risk is set up to ask a question that is not important or has already been answered by previous research, the risk/benefit profile is likely to be unfavorable. The point is that the IRB is obligated to evaluate the study design and other aspects of scientific quality because these are ethical issues that affect the rights and welfare of research participants.

When Study Design Is Suboptimal but Risk Is Minimal

Having stressed the importance of evaluating the scientific quality of research, it is important to remember that as with all ethical principles, the IRB should use judgment and common sense when considering the rejection of a study based on problems with the study design. In organizations where a large volume of social science research is done by students, it is not unusual for the IRB to review protocols where the scientific design is not optimal but the risk to subjects is virtually zero.

Although one could argue that many of these student projects could be classified as educational exercises rather than research, that is a separate issue. The point is that there are projects where the study design is flawed, but the risk is basically zero. Certainly, it makes sense for IRB members who are knowledgeable in the research to recommend revisions to the study plan. However, in the absence of risk, there is no strong ethical justification for the IRB to make revisions a condition for IRB approval. The IRB may choose to address issues of this nature, for example in student research, in ways other than voting against one particular protocol; for example, it might initiate a dialog with the department chairperson or program leader.

REFERENCES

Nuremberg Code. (1947). From "Trials of War Criminals Before the Nuremberg Military Tribunals Under Control Council Law No. 10," Vol. 2. (Washington, DC: U.S. Government Printing Office, 1949), pp. 181–182. Available: http://ohsr.od.nih.gov/guidelines/nuremberg.html.

Protection of Human Subjects, 45 C. F. R. pt. 46 (2009).

World Medical Association. *Declaration of Helsinki: Ethical principles for research involving human subjects.* As amended in Seoul, 2008. Available: http://www.wma.net/en/30publications/10policies/b3/17c.pdf (accessed February 3, 2010).

Researcher Conflict of Interest

Daniel K. Nelson and Robert Amdur

Researcher Conflict of Interest

- For the purposes of IRB determinations, we can define a *conflict of interest* as a set of conditions in which an investigator's judgment concerning a primary interest (e.g., subject's welfare, integrity of research) may be biased by a secondary interest (e.g., personal gain).
- Saying that a conflict of interest exists does not mean that somebody made the wrong decision. It means that people who evaluate the situation may reasonably conclude that the potential for bias is such that improper decisions are possible.
- Disclosure to subjects does not, in and of itself, make a conflict of interest acceptable. Ethical research requires both disclosure *and* effective management of conflicts of interest.
- The IRB has several options for managing investigator conflict of interest, including the following:
  Prohibit conflicted investigators from having any involvement in the study.
  Prohibit conflicted investigators from participating in key components of the study—for example, the consent process, evaluation of inclusion criteria, specific procedures, and overall data analysis.
  Require a person who is not connected in any way to the investigator or study sponsor to act as a subject advocate during the initial and ongoing consent process.

Conflicts of interest are inherent to the conduct of research. In 1978, the National Commission for the Protection of Human Subjects of Biomedical and Behavioral Research, as it deliberated toward the Belmont Report, wrote that "investigators are always in positions of potential conflict by virtue of their concern with the pursuit of knowledge as well as the welfare of the human subjects of their research." The commission echoed earlier reports by the NIH and the surgeon general in viewing investigators as poorly positioned to reconcile these competing interests on their own, and in calling for a shared responsibility that incorporated independent review, such as the IRB. The National Bioethics Advisory Commission (NBAC) reiterated this fundamental observation more than 20 years later when it examined our system of protections, noting that research "necessarily creates a conflict of interest for investigators" (2001, p. 11) through their use of fellow humans to obtain knowledge. Note that neither commission held these conflicts to be irreconcilable, nor did they link conflict of interest to character flaws of investigators, as individuals or as a class. The goals of this chapter are to define conflict of interest and to discuss possible management strategies.

DEFINITIONS

Before considering conflicts of interest as they relate to research involving human subjects, it is important to establish a working definition. One source of confusion lies in the semantics of the discussion. The problem that we are trying to avoid is *bias in judgment.* We are looking for a term to describe situations where the potential for bias is such that decisions may be called into question. For the purposes of IRB determinations, a *conflict of interest* can be defined as a set of conditions in which an investigator's judgment concerning a primary interest (e.g., subject's welfare, integrity of research) may be biased by a secondary interest (e.g., personal gain).

One of the most misunderstood aspects of conflict of interest is that a problem exists even in the absence of documentation of bias or improper decisions. Saying that a conflict of interest exists does not mean that somebody made the wrong decision. It means that people who evaluate the situation may reasonably conclude that the potential for bias is such that improper decisions are likely. In other words, it is the people who evaluate the decision, not the person making the decisions, who determine if a conflict of interest exists. P. J. Friedman explains, "A conflict exists whether or not decisions are affected by the personal interest; a conflict of interest implies only the potential for bias or wrongdoing, not a certainty or likelihood" (1992, pp. 245–251).

With regard to financial relationships, former *New England Journal of Medicine* editor Marcia Angell has defined conflict of interest as "any financial association that would cause an investigator to prefer one outcome . . . to another" (2000). Angell argues that there is no such thing as potential conflict of interest, because conflict is a function of the situation, not of the investigator's response to that situation. Thus the opportunity need not be acted on to represent a conflict of interest and a situation worthy of concern.

DISCLOSURE

In 1914 Supreme Court Justice Louis Brandeis wrote that "publicity is justly commended as a remedy for social and industrial diseases. Sunlight is said to be the best of disinfectants" (Brandeis University, n.d.).

Disclosure to the Institution

Disclosure to the institution is mandatory for those investigators receiving federal funds, with their institutions given discretion in how they manage any conflicts. Predictably, there is considerable variability in how institutions handle this process. Many have established policies requiring disclosure by all faculty members. However, few institutions have linked this process to protection of human subjects, as suggested by the fact that none of the 235 institutions in a recent survey incorporated disclosure to either IRBs or subjects as a management strategy in their conflict of interest policies.

Disclosure to the IRB

Disclosure to the IRB is increasingly advocated as a routine part of protocol review. OHRP has strongly recommended that financial relationships be described when investigators submit IRB applications, and that IRBs should take into consideration the funding arrangements between sponsor and investigator institution. A recent survey of 200 IRBs that oversee clinical trials suggests that only 25% review such financial matters. These have tended to be regarded, by both investigators and IRBs, as none of their business. However, if IRBs are to fulfill their responsibility to protect research subjects from bias related to conflict of interest, they must evaluate the financial and other incentives that motivate the conduct of studies they review.

Disclosure to Subjects

Disclosure via the informed consent process is at once the most direct and ethically intuitive route of disclosure, but also the most difficult to accomplish in a meaningful way. At the very least, subjects should be aware that the study is sponsored by outside entities, be they commercial or governmental. As to the level of detail provided, we stop short of recommending that consent forms routinely include dollar amounts, even when investigators are paid on a per capita basis. Dollar amounts may be misleading, because some may represent justifiable expenses, some may represent inappropriate incentives, and some are both at the same time.

A major misunderstanding for IRBs and investigators is the concept that full disclosure to subjects makes a conflict of interest acceptable. This is not the case. Ethical research requires both disclosure *and* effective management of conflicts of interest. IRBs must not pass the buck to subjects by shirking their responsibility to evaluate the possibility that conflicts will bias judgments in the conduct or analysis of research. It is well documented that research subjects often do not understand this kind of information beyond a superficial level. The principle of beneficence requires that the IRB not approve a study when there is a conflict of interest that is likely to bias judgment to a meaningful degree, regardless of the extent to which the conflict is explained in the consent process.

BEYOND DISCLOSURE

Management strategies should be aimed at eliminating or minimizing the conflict of interest. Although IRBs may not be well situated or equipped to directly oversee this process, they should establish open lines of communication with those institutional bodies that are better situated (e.g., the conflict of interest committee). IRBs should then consider the mechanisms proposed to manage the identified conflict, with a particular eye for aspects that could affect research subjects. The IRB has several options for managing investigator conflict of interest in the context of a given study:

- Prohibit conflicted investigators from having any involvement in the study.
- Prohibit conflicted investigators from participating in key components of the study—for example, the consent process, evaluation of inclusion criteria, specific procedures, and overall data analysis.
- Require a person who is not connected in any way to the investigator or study sponsor to act as a subject advocate during the initial and ongoing consent process.

Given that even the appearance of impropriety is enough to damage individual careers and institutional reputations, a cautious approach to these issues is in everyone's mutual interest. IRBs may first need to overcome the perception that managing conflict of interest is reliant on their trust of the investigator in question. Management should hinge not on anyone's perception of an individual but on an objective assessment of situations in which people have placed themselves. All parties involved in this process should be clear that managing conflict of interest has everything to do with the situation and nothing to do with the character or honesty of the individual under question.

REFERENCES

Angell, M. (2000, August). *Plenary: Reaction to conference proceedings.* Panel presented at Conference on Human Subject Protection and Financial Conflicts of Interest, Bethesda, MD. Transcript retrieved from http://www.hhs.gov/ohrp/coi/8-16.htm#Angell.

Brandeis University. (n.d.) *Louis D. Brandeis Legacy Fund for Social Justice: Biography.* Available: http://www.brandeis.edu/legacyfund /bio.html.

Friedman, P. J. (1992). The troublesome semantics of conflict of interest. *Ethics and Behavior, 2*(4), 245–251.

National Bioethics Advisory Commission. (2001). *Ethical and policy issues in research involving human participants.* Bethesda, MD: Author. Available: http://www.bioethics.gov/reports/past _commissions/nbac_human_part.pdf.

National Commission for the Protection of Human Subjects of Biomedical and Behavioral Research. (1979). *Belmont Report.* Available: http://www.hhs.gov/ohrp/humansubjects/guidance /belmont.htm.

IRB Member Conflict of Interest

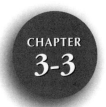

CHAPTER
3-3

Daniel K. Nelson

Sources of IRB Conflict of Interest

Individual Level

- Member is investigator on research under review
- Members or staff hold significant financial interest in sponsor of research
- Loyalty to colleagues submitting for review
- Members closely tied to area of research under review
  Familiar = too lenient
  Competitor = too critical
- Possible impact of decisions on member's own work (e.g., policy changes)
- Personal agendas or advocacy positions
- Non-IRB roles of members
  Contracts and grants office
  Legal counsel

Institutional Level

- Pressure or desire to protect the institution
- Concern for institution's reputation or prestige
- Promoting research vs. protecting subjects
- Undervaluation of IRB service
- Potential liability
- Institutional or community values
- Pressure for speedy reviews
- Institutional equity or ownership
- Review fees

Given the central role of IRBs in overseeing the ethical conduct of research involving human subjects, it is critical that they operate free from inappropriate influence. Accordingly, IRB members, chairpersons, and staff should follow policies and procedures similar to those of investigators to eliminate or manage any conflicts of interest. In this context, a conflict of interest can be defined as any situation or relationship that biases, or has the potential to bias, the conduct or outcome of IRB review.

SOURCES OF IRB CONFLICT OF INTEREST: INDIVIDUAL LEVEL

Research by IRB Members

Perhaps the most widely recognized conflict of interest for IRBs is when research conducted by one of the members comes up for review. The investigator-member has an obvious interest in seeing the research approved for a number of personal and professional reasons. Because this type of conflict is usually apparent, proper management is largely a procedural matter. Beyond this direct conflict involving review of members' own research, there are multiple sources for indirect conflict of interest. These may be harder to discern and, therefore, harder to manage.

IRB Members' Financial Interests

One example of these less apparent conflicts is a situation where an IRB member or staff person holds significant equity or other financial interests in the research itself or in the sponsors of research. These might include equity holdings, consulting arrangements, or patent rights—in short, the same types of financial conflicts that investigators might hold. Although the majority of academic research institutions have policies governing financial conflicts of interest, these invariably focus on faculty serving as investigators and not as IRB members. The same concerns would apply, however, regarding the objectivity of individuals who stand to gain financially from research they are being asked to review and approve.

Loyalty to Colleagues

Another potential source of conflict is loyalty to colleagues submitting research for IRB review—be they peers, subordinates, or superiors. Members might logically be inclined to support the work of departmental colleagues with whom they interact every day (i.e., more directly than with other IRB members). Beyond mere camaraderie, members may sense a need to promote the work of subordinates or to avoid antagonizing their chief with a critical review. At a practical level, this conflict may be impossible to avoid because few institutions are large enough to assemble a panel of individuals with sufficient insight who do not also have overlapping interactions with colleagues submitting research.

Members' Areas of Expertise

Selection of members with sufficient expertise to comprehend the complexities of the research under review presents another potential problem. Members whose training or own area of research is closely tied to the studies under review may tend to show more leniency than they might to other areas with which they are less familiar. That is, it may be natural for them to take novel issues or procedures for granted. Conversely, this familiarity might work in the opposite direction if reviewers regard submitting investigators as competitors or rivals and are more critical than they might be otherwise. Members in this position might also find themselves with access to proprietary information when reviewing protocols, providing tempting insight to ongoing research in their personal area of interest. Whether overly lenient or overly critical, neither tendency is conducive to the objective review that the IRB should strive to achieve.

Impact of Decisions

IRB members might also be mindful of the possible impact of IRB decisions on their own work. For example, an IRB member who does clinical outcome studies may be reluctant to support IRB decisions that strengthen privacy protection if these lead to policies that restrict his or her own access to medical records for research.

Personal Agendas

Personal agendas of members may also interfere with the review process. For example, members of an advocacy group for a given disease or disorder can yield valuable insight as community representatives but can represent a negative influence if they see their role as promoting a certain agenda.

Non-IRB Roles

The institutional roles filled by members in their daily work outside the IRB may carry inherent conflicts of interest. For example, the director of a university contracts and grants office, whose primary duties revolve around bringing more research support into the institution, may not be an appropriate individual to serve on the IRB. The same could be said for any institutional official charged with promoting or supporting the research enterprise if that obligation might run counter to a critical assessment of protocols. Indeed, reliance on individuals with these types of position conflicts has been cited as an unacceptable situation in recent federal compliance actions. Another institutional role that may exclude a person from IRB service is that of the legal counsel. Although legal counsel can be extremely helpful in an advisory capacity, a primary role of protecting the institution may run counter to the IRB's mission of protecting the subject. It can be argued that these goals are not incompatible to the extent that a happy subject is a happy institution, but care must be exercised to avoid conflicting objectives.

The preceding discussion should not detract from the clear benefit of having IRB members with legal training, which is increasingly important for interpreting and applying regulations, interdigitating with state laws, and multiple other functions. Similarly, members with insight on the financing of research can provide valuable input to IRB deliberations. Nevertheless, care should be taken when appointing members who will be forced to wear too many institutional hats in serving the IRB.

SOURCES OF CONFLICT OF INTEREST:
INSTITUTIONAL LEVEL

Protecting the Institution

Apart from any internal desire to protect the institution on the part of individual members, the institution must also avoid placing external pressure on the IRB to serve in this role. This may be a natural expectation for deans, provosts, presidents, and other officials and, as previously mentioned, is not necessarily incompatible with the role of the IRB, but should never be confused with its primary role. This separation of roles will be especially important as penalties for noncompliance continue to increase and institutions come to view their IRBs as a chief means of preventing regulatory sanctions.

Enhancing the Institution

In a more positive direction, a related source of conflict could arise from members' innate concerns for their institution's reputation or prestige, to the extent that this is enhanced through an active research portfolio. Once again, this desire is not incompatible with sound IRB review, but it should never be an excuse for relaxing standards in the review of research.

Promoting Research

Yet another related concern is the desire on the part of individual members—and on the part of the IRB as an agent of the institution—to promote research in general. This is a laudable goal, but it should never be pursued to the extent that it detracts from the IRB's reason for being, which is to protect the rights and welfare of human subjects.

Value of Membership

Undervaluation of service to the IRB is another factor that could translate into a conflict of interest. If members do not believe that their work on the IRB is appreciated or valued by their superiors, they may not believe that they can or should devote the time necessary to do the job well. Department chairpersons, deans, and other institutional officials should send a clear signal that IRB membership is a necessary and important activity and recognize such service when considering promotions, tenure, and clinical work schedules. Some institutions are going beyond this by compensating home departments for the time faculty spend on IRB duties.

Liability

The potential for legal liability is another factor that could influence an IRB's decision making. Although lawsuits implicating the IRB have been relatively few in number, and most institutions are likely to indemnify IRB members in the performance of their professional duties, the threat of lawsuit is an ever-present possibility in our litigious society. Possible sources of lawsuits include not only subjects who have been injured in research, but also investigators who believe their research has been unfairly hindered by an IRB.

Institutional or Community Values

Institutional or community values are another source of possible conflict to the extent they may be reflected in reviews by individual members or the IRB as a whole. Clearly there is a regulatory mandate that the IRB reflect community attitudes, but there may be times when these values run counter to the mission of the IRB. For example, some institutions may be particularly sensitive to social or political issues (e.g., abortion) in ways that run counter to regulatory guidance that IRBs should not consider the long-range public policy implications of research under review. This separation from institutional values may admittedly be difficult to achieve when beliefs are deeply held.

Pressure for Speed

IRB members or staff often come under pressure from individual investigators or from the institution to conduct a speedy review. Although it may be in everyone's best interest to establish systems for review that are both effective and efficient, the process should not be hastened to the point that important issues are overlooked.

Institutional Holdings or Interests

Institutions are increasingly entering agreements with industry that may create conflict of interest for the institution. These arrangements might include patent rights for new innovations, spin-off companies, technology licensing, or equity holdings. If an institution will be conducting research in which it bears a direct financial interest, appropriate firewalls should be in place to ensure that ethical oversight (i.e., the IRB) is not subject to influence from the institution. If the independence of the IRB cannot be assured, it may be preferable to solicit the services of another IRB or to conduct the research at other institutions.

Review Fees

Finally, the charging of review fees may create a conflict of interest that biases IRB review. Institutions that compete successfully for federal grant support receive a sizable percentage in the form of indirect costs, which are intended to support a variety of functions necessary to conduct research. Many institutions, perhaps now the majority, have begun charging review fees for industry-sponsored protocols as a means of generating additional support for the IRB. These fees, ranging from a few hundred to a few thousand dollars, are legitimate sources of revenue for work performed. All parties should be clear, however, that the fees are linked to protocol submissions and are not contingent on approval by the IRB. It is also highly advisable that the fees be administered through mechanisms separate from the IRB (e.g., contracts and grants office, billing department, or other administrative entities), so that the IRB is not placed in the position of bill collector. Ideally, the IRB should operate in complete ignorance of the billing status of any individual protocol. This also presents a conflict for independent, for-profit IRBs, which may derive their entire revenue from such fees. There is nothing inherently improper in this arrangement, and many independent IRBs conduct credible, ethical review. They are, however, subject to an added element of conflict because they are businesses in their own right. This makes them dependent on the good will and satisfaction of their clients (e.g., pharmaceutical companies or contract research organizations), who are free to take their business elsewhere. This might logically occur if reviews were consistently perceived as being nit-picky, unfavorable, or slow. Thus, independent IRBs may be subject to conflict of interest pressures over and above those facing institution-based IRBs. Conversely, it can be argued that independent IRBs are free from many of the influences discussed previously because they are not subject to institutional expectations and pressures. Each setting will have its own set of motivating factors, and neither is free from conflicts of interest.

REGULATORY GUIDANCE

If the IRB is to function in an independent, unbiased manner, it must not be subject to inappropriate pressures. Recognizing this, federal regulations specifically addressed IRB conflict of interest long before investigator conflict of interest became a focus of regulatory guidance. Both HHS3[Sec.107(e)] and FDA4[Sec.107(e)] regulations instruct that "no IRB may have a member participate in the IRB's initial or continuing review of any project in which the member has a conflicting interest, except to provide information requested by the IRB." This means that each IRB should have clearly defined mechanisms for identifying conflicts among its members and for excluding conflicted members from a situation where review may be compromised.

MANAGEMENT OF IRB CONFLICTS OF INTEREST

In contrast to the enormous attention paid to investigator conflicts of interest in recent years, very little has been paid to similar conflicts on the part of IRBs. This may be partly because IRBs are not involved hands-on with the actual conduct of the study, and partly because those involved with ethical review are seen as somehow immune to baser instincts. For whatever reason, few authors or policy makers have specifically addressed the conflicts that might be faced by IRBs or their resolution. As with conflicts for investigators, the first (and perhaps most difficult) task is to recognize that a conflict exists. Once this conflict is identified and acknowledged, steps should be taken to eliminate or minimize its impact. For the purpose of discussion, let us consider the fairly routine scenario where an IRB member is involved as an investigator on the research under review, recognizing that many of the conflicts described earlier in this chapter might be addressed through similar mechanisms. As with identification of conflicts for the larger pool of investigators outside the IRB, this process would typically rely on self-identification by the investigator-member. Once conflicts are identified, written policies and procedures should describe how the conflicted member will be removed from deliberations on the protocol for which he or she holds the conflict.

Recusal of Members From Meetings

In the setting of a convened meeting, the most obvious solution is that the member in question should physically leave the room during consideration of any protocol in which he or she has a conflict of interest. This approach minimizes two sources of influence—neither of them desirable. First, the investigator-member would naturally be inclined to give the protocol preferential treatment. Second, other members may not feel completely free to discuss openly or to criticize out of deference to their fellow board member. Thus, removal from the meeting is the clearest means by which to manage that member's conflict. Some IRBs, however, wish the member to remain present for initial discussion to answer any questions, just as they would want any other investigator to do. As noted previously, this is expressly allowed by the regulations. If an IRB chooses to adopt this as local policy, remaining members should be given further opportunity for discussion once the conflicted member eventually does leave the meeting.

In some circumstances, the IRB may be placed in an untenable position if the physical absence of a conflicted member would force the loss of quorum, thereby halting the meeting. This creates a catch-22 of sorts if the IRB would prefer that any conflicted member leave the room, yet needs that member present in order to meet regulatory requirements for quorum. Under these circumstances, one would hope that the valid concept of having sufficient numbers present to conduct business (i.e., a quorum) would give way to the intent behind these regulatory requirements, namely, to ensure that research undergoes review by an unbiased, independent body.

This author's personal opinion is that we may be missing the forest for the trees if it means compromising review by keeping a conflicted member present only to preserve an arbitrary quorum. This argument gains more credence when we remember that the minimum quorum under existing regulations requires that only 3 members be present (of the minimum 5 total members), and that most IRBs are much larger than that in practice, even at half strength. That is, one could envision a situation where an IRB with 20 members had 11 members in attendance and wished to temporarily excuse a conflicted member. It is difficult to accept that the remaining 10 members are insufficient to conduct review, when 10 still represents thrice the number required for a duly constituted quorum under regulatory requirements.

All that said, the regulations do require the presence of a quorum, and the foregoing is not an argument to disregard that requirement. The best approach is to ensure that adequate numbers of members will be present so that quorum is never endangered. This can be accomplished through the use of alternates to cover absences, reminders on the days of meetings, and selection of members who will take seriously their commitment to attend.

Conclusion

Any conflicts of interest on the part of the IRB undermine the credibility of the process and must be avoided at all costs. Whether a particular influence is real or perceived, originates from within or without, or is felt consciously or subconsciously, IRBs are not immune from conflicts of interest. No one doubts the integrity or motivation of those serving to protect human subjects, but IRBs are no more or less human than the investigators they oversee, and they can only benefit from self-awareness in areas that might impact their effectiveness.

Advertisements for Research

RACHEL HOMER, RACHEL KREBS, AND LINDA MEDWAR

Advertisements for Research

The IRB must approve all plans for advertisement (including the actual posters, brochures, scripts for commercials, etc.) prior to their use. A 1998 update of the FDA information sheet, *Recruiting Study Subjects,* presents the following guidelines for the format of study advertisement:

- Name and address of the investigator and/or research facility/institution
- Condition under study and/or purpose of the research
- Inclusion/exclusion criteria in summary form
- A brief list of procedures involved
- Time or other commitment required (number of visits, total duration including follow-up visits, etc.)
- Compensation/reimbursement
- Location of research and contact person for further information

Additional guidelines include the following:

- Advertisements should not emphasize monetary compensation.
- Advertisements should not use catchy words like *free* or *exciting.*
- Advertisements should be very clear that *research* participation is what is being solicited.
- Advertisements should not be misleading about the purpose of the research.

The recruitment of subjects, which is considered the start of the consent/assent process, and the feasibility of recruiting must be considered and planned before initiation of a study and must continue throughout the study. For this reason, the IRB must review the methods, materials, procedures, and tools used to recruit potential research subjects before they are implemented. Some of the more commonly used tools of recruitment include direct advertising (flyers, posters, press releases, brochures), media advertisements (newspaper, TV, radio, websites), recruitment letters, review of medical charts and computerized databases, and presentations at community meeting places.

FLYERS, POSTERS, AND BROCHURES

Flyers, posters, and brochures are often used to solicit potential research subjects. These types of advertisements are typically placed in strategic locations in the hope of targeting the population being studied. Some of these locations may include bulletin boards, professional offices/businesses, schools, public transportation vehicles (buses, subways, trains), and public areas such as restaurants. Although it is mandatory to obtain IRB approval for use of such advertisements, it may also be necessary for an investigator to obtain approval from the various sites where the flyer, poster, and/or brochure will be placed. This should also be done prior to posting or distribution of the ad, and evidence of this approval may be required by the IRB. Because these types of advertisements are visible tools of recruitment, they must present sufficient information that is accurate and balanced so that potential subjects are able to make an informed decision about possible participation. The decision to include compensation and/or reimbursement in the advertisement may be made on a case-by-case basis, depending on the study itself and the particular policies and guidelines of the IRB. Although compensation or reimbursement may factor into one's decision to participate in a study, its mention in advertisements must be carefully thought out and worded appropriately so as not to coerce a subject to participate. The examples of acceptable and unacceptable research advertisements presented here will clarify these issues.

Figure 3-4.1 presents an advertisement that should not be approved by the IRB. Several problems can be seen in this advertisement, including:

- Monetary compensation is emphasized.
- Catchy words such as *exciting, fast, cutting-edge,* and *free* are used.
- The ages for eligibility are not specified.
- The purpose of the study is not specified.
- There is no mention that this study is for research.
- Terms such as *fat* may be insulting.
- The name of contact person is not included.
- The study location is not included.
- The purpose of the advertisement is misleading.

Figure 3-4.2 is an advertisement that meets the basic guidelines for IRB approval, including:

- The approach is straightforward and honest.
- The type of research is specified.
- The ages for eligibility are included.
- The purpose is clearly stated.

Figure 3-4.1 Unapproved Advertisement

LOSE WEIGHT FAST AND RECEIVE CASH!!!
JOIN AN EXCITING WEIGHT LOSS STUDY

- *Are you a teenager?*
- *Are you fat, and do you want to lose weight?*

If you answered YES to these questions, you may qualify to participate in a weight loss study.

You will receive a **free** medical evaluation and participate in a cutting-edge nutrition program. You will also receive $$$ money $$$ and parking vouchers. No medications will be given.

Call (213) 456-9870 for more information.

- The benefits are included.
- The contact person's name is included.
- The institution is identified.

Figure 3-4.2 Revised Advertisement

> ***WEIGHT LOSS AND DIABETES PREVENTION STUDY***
> ***BE PART OF AN IMPORTANT NUTRITION RESEARCH STUDY***
>
> - *Are you between 13 and 21 years of age?*
> - *Do you want to change your eating habits in order to lose weight?*
>
> If you answered **YES** to these questions, you may be eligible to participate in a nutrition research study.
>
> The purpose of this research study is to compare the effectiveness of different diets in preventing Type 2 diabetes. Benefits include a comprehensive medical evaluation and nutrition program. Participants will also receive monetary compensation and parking vouchers. No medications will be given.
>
> Both **adolescents** (13 years of age and older) and **adults** (21 years of age and younger) are eligible.
>
> The study is being conducted at Central Hospital.
>
> **Please call Beth Woods at**
> **(213) 456-9870 for more information.**

Paying Research Subjects

BRUCE G. GORDON, JOSEPH BROWN,
CHRISTOPHER KRATOCHVIL,
ERNEST D. PRENTICE, AND ROBERT AMDUR

Paying Research Subjects

- Determining reimbursement versus inducement is the first step in evaluating the ethics of payment of research subjects.
- Reimbursement does not include payment for taking risks or experiencing discomfort or inconvenience.
- Reimbursing subjects for expenses that they actually incur as a result of research participation seems a minimum reasonable approach.
- If the IRB decides that inducement payments are acceptable, there are two basic models for determining the appropriate level of payment—the market model and the wage payment model.

Paying subjects to participate in research remains one of the most contentious ethical problems for IRBs. This chapter will review the practice and review some practical approaches.

REIMBURSEMENT VERSUS INDUCEMENT

To evaluate the ethics of paying subjects for their participation in research, the first thing the IRB should do is determine if the payment is a reimbursement or an inducement. A payment is a reimbursement when it is meant to directly offset the direct, out-of-pocket costs that a subject incurs as a result of participating in the study. In contrast to a reimbursement, an inducement is a payment that is meant to motivate the subject to participate in the study for financial gain.

The distinction between reimbursement and inducement payments is critical to the IRB evaluation process. We find no ethical controversy to reimbursements for costs related to research participation regardless of the dollar amount of the payment. By definition, reimbursements do not coerce people into participating in research. Inducement payments are what the IRB should worry about, and it is this category of payment that the IRB must struggle with as it tries to determine where appropriate compensation ends and undue inducement begins.

Ethical Arguments Regarding Inducement Payments for Research Participation

Inducement Payments and Undue Influence

The main argument against using money to induce people to participate in research is that such payments represent undue influence. Undue influence violates the Belmont principle of respect for persons, which requires that research participation be completely voluntary. Financial inducements may (and indeed are designed to) get people to do something they would not otherwise do (e.g., participate in research). The counterargument is that it is paternalistic for the IRB to prevent subjects from doing something that they want to do as long as they understand the implications of their decision.

Inducement Payments and the Belmont Principle of Justice

Another argument against inducement payments is that they violate the Belmont principle of justice because such payments may result in economically disadvantaged persons bearing a disproportionately large share of the risks of research. The counterargument is that research should not be considered solely as a burden. To the extent that the benefits of research are distributed primarily to participants, one might argue that any procedure such as payment of subjects that encourages recruitment of populations that have traditionally not participated in clinical research, like African Americans, is ethically acceptable and appropriate.

MODELS FOR PAYMENT

IRBs that ultimately decide to allow payment to research subjects must decide what level of compensation is appropriate. The literature on this subject describes the following three common models for paying research subjects: (1) market model, (2) wage payment model, and (3) reimbursement model.

Market Model

In the market model, the laws of supply and demand determine how much a subject should be paid for participating in a given trial. The payment level is determined primarily by the trade-off between the potential risks and benefits of research participation with the highest payments going to subjects who accept a high level of risk or discomfort relative to expected benefit. This model also allows for higher compensation to speed recruitment and bonuses to ensure that subjects complete the study.

Wage Payment Model

In this model, payment is made based on the premise that participation in research is unskilled labor that requires little training and some risk. Thus, subjects are compensated on a scale commensurate with that of other unskilled but essential jobs—that is, a fairly low, standardized hourly wage, with bonuses for hazardous procedures.

Reimbursement Model

The reimbursement model will be the model of choice for the IRB member who decides that inducement payments of any amount are unacceptable. In the reimbursement model, payment is equal to the expenses that the subject actually incurred as a result of participating in the research study. The definition of *expenses* may be flexible and can include lost wages resulting from time taken off from work without pay. The reimbursement model does not compensate subjects for inconvenience or discomfort.

OTHER ISSUES CONCERNING PAYMENT

Prorating Payment

The FDA clearly requires a system of prorating payments based on the duration of participation of the subject in the research. The FDA information sheets state, "Any credit for payment should accrue as the study progresses and not be contingent upon the subject completing the entire study" (2009). Prorated payment should be made regardless of whether withdrawal was voluntary or involuntary.

Payment to Minors

Though the majority of IRBs allow payment of children who participate in research, there is limited and sometimes conflicting guidance from regulatory agencies and professional organizations. Certainly the same ethical concerns that affect payment of adults apply to minors as subjects, but the issues appear more complicated. Children and adolescents may be more or less prone to being unduly influenced by financial reward, depending on their age and maturity. Children and younger adolescents often have limited capability to understand the risks and, therefore, are not likely to perform an adequate assessment of the risk–benefit relationship. This may be especially true for adolescents, who feel invulnerable and indestructible, and therefore may be especially prey to monetary inducements.

If payment to the child is concerning, payment to the parent is also ethically problematic. The American Academy of Pediatrics notes that "serious ethical questions arise when payment is offered to adults acting on behalf of minors in return for allowing minors to participate as research subjects" (1995). However, it could be argued that payment to the parent is preferable because the parent (rather than the child) incurs the financial costs of participating in research (e.g., loss of wages, car expenses, food).

The best compromise may be a combination of payments: reimbursement for financial costs of research participation to the parents and as some remuneration to the child who is bearing the burden of research. When paying minors directly, a good guideline is to make payment equal to the minimum hourly wage.

Lotteries

As an added complication to the issue of compensation, occasionally the IRB receives a request to allow the use of a lottery or raffle (of money or goods) as a form of subject compensation, or as a method of encouraging participation in research. Subject participation in the lottery may occur upon enrollment in the study or may be contingent upon compliance with the protocol and completion of the study.

Use of a lottery presents additional ethical concerns. It has been argued that lotteries violate the principle of justice because of the unequal distribution of something of value—namely, that only one person wins the lottery. Second, given that most people overvalue their likelihood to win a lottery, the offering of a large payment serves to undermine the process of informed consent. Because this overvaluing is greatest when chances to win are small, lotteries with large prizes and small probabilities of winning are particularly problematic. Finally, no study is entirely free of costs, and those studies with small costs ought to have correspondingly small compensation. Payment of large prizes to a very small number of participants violates this balance of subject participation and compensation, creating serious concerns about undue inducements to participation.

REFERENCES

American Academy of Pediatrics, Committee on Drugs. (1995). Guidelines for the ethical conduct of studies to evaluate drugs in pediatric populations. *Pediatrics, 95*(2), 286–294.

U.S. Food and Drug Administration. (2009). *Payment to research subjects.* Available: http://www.fda.gov/ScienceResearch/Special Topics/RunningClinicalTrials/GuidancesInformationSheetsand Notices/ucm116330.htm.

Denying Subjects Access to Research Results

THOMAS KEENS AND ROBERT AMDUR

Denying Subjects Access to Research Results

- Ethical research requires that subjects understand the conditions under which they will, or will not, be given research results.
- When considering the ethics of withholding research results from subjects, the important questions are the predictive value of the research result and the potential social or psychological harm subjects may experience as a result of being given this type of speculative information.
- In some situations, it is appropriate for the research plan to deny subjects access to research results.
- When subjects may experience serious psychological distress from reviewing a research result, the study plan should include professional counseling to minimize the risk of study participation.

When research involves testing of subjects for potential markers of disease, the IRB must evaluate the plans of the study for informing the subjects of research results. Some studies plan to give subjects research results whether they ask for them or not, whereas others give subjects results only in specific situations.

ETHICAL PRINCIPLES

The Belmont principles of respect for persons and beneficence address the issue of informing subjects about research results. At first glance, these principles appear to present competing obligations.

Respect for Persons

Respect for persons means that ethical research requires subjects to understand the full implications of their decision to participate in a study. There are two ways one could apply the principle of respect for persons to the question of informing subjects of research results. One view is that respect for persons requires that researchers give each subject the option of being informed of research results, with a full explanation of the potential implications of this decision. The alternative view is that the principle of respect for persons requires that potential subjects understand whether they will or will not be informed of research results, but that that there is no ethical justification for requiring result disclosure. Subjects are not required to participate in research. It is perfectly ethical to allow people to exercise their right as autonomous agents to decline to participate in a research study because they do not agree with the plan to limit access to research results.

Beneficence

Beneficence includes the obligation to maximize potential benefits and minimize potential risks. This principle means that investigators should provide every subject with research information if that information will maximize benefits or minimize risks to the subject. But the principle of beneficence also means that the investigator should not inform the subject about research results if that information will cause harm.

There are situations where informing a subject about research results will cause psychological distress, stigmatization, discrimination, or other forms of social harm. This usual situation when it could be harmful to inform subjects about a research result is when the meaning of the result in unclear. With speculative information—meaning information that has not been proved to have clinical relevance—the principle of beneficence suggests that the investigator is not obligated to inform the research subject of research results.

RECOMMENDATIONS

As part of the review of human research protocols, IRBs must decide whether or not research information should be given to subjects. To help in this determination, the IRB should consider the following issues:

1. A complete understanding of the extent to which research results will be disclosed to the subjects is an absolute requirement of ethical research.

2. When considering the ethics of withholding research results from subjects, the important questions are the predictive value of the research result and the potential social or psychological harm subjects may experience as a result of being given this type of speculative information.

3. In some situations, it is appropriate for the research plan to deny subjects access to research results.

4. When subjects may experience serious psychological distress from reviewing a research result, the study plan should include professional counseling to minimize the risk of study participation.

Deception
of Research
Subjects

CHAPTER
3-7

LAURIE SLONE, JAY HULL, AND ROBERT AMDUR

Deception of Research Subjects

The American Psychological Association (APA) has developed guidelines for the conduct of research that involves deception of subjects:

- Psychologists never deceive research participants about significant aspects that would affect their willingness to participate, such as physical risks, discomfort, or unpleasant emotional experiences.
- Any other deception that is an integral feature of the design and conduct of an experiment must be explained to participants as early as is feasible—preferably, at the conclusion of their participation, but no later than at the conclusion of the research.

PROVIDING PARTICIPANTS WITH INFORMATION ABOUT THE STUDY

- If scientific or humane values justify delaying or withholding this information, psychologists take reasonable measures to reduce the risk of harm.

The following guidelines should be applied to the consent document:

- The consent document should never be used as part of the deception and thus should not include anything that is untrue.

continues

Deception of Research Subjects *continued*

- The consent document should reveal as much as possible to the participant regarding the procedures in the study.
- The consent document need not explain the details of the study if this will eliminate the capability of the study to inform the process under investigation.

The purpose of this chapter is to discuss research in which the subject is intentionally deceived about research participation. Deception is common in studies that evaluate human behavior. The rationale for deception in this setting is that it is not possible to obtain accurate information about how people behave when they know that their behavior is being evaluated.

GUIDELINES FOR RESEARCH INVOLVING DECEPTION

If one grants that it is impossible to study certain aspects of human behavior without adopting deceptive techniques, then the justification of such research evolves into a question of costs and benefits—the benefits gained by knowledge relative to the potential harm caused by deception. To some extent, this is a question of personal values. However, it also suggests that specific codes of conduct should be developed that serve to minimize the negative impact of deceptive techniques. The APA has developed such a code. The two sections relevant to deception in research read as follows:

8.07 Deception in Research

a. Psychologists do not conduct a study involving deception unless they have determined that the use of deceptive techniques is justified by the study's significant prospective scientific, educational, or applied value and that equally effective non-deceptive alternative procedures are not feasible.

b. Psychologists do not deceive prospective participants about research that is reasonably expected to cause physical pain or severe emotional distress.

c. Psychologists explain any deception that is an integral feature of the design and conduct of an experiment to participants as early as is feasible, preferably at the conclusion of their participation, but no later than at the conclusion of the data collection, and permit participants to withdraw their data. (APA, 2002)

8.02 Providing Participants with Information about the Study

a. Psychologists provide a prompt opportunity for participants to obtain appropriate information about the nature, results, and conclusions of the research, and they take reasonable steps to correct any misconceptions that participants may have of which the psychologists are aware.

b. If scientific or humane values justify delaying or withholding this information, psychologists take reasonable measures to reduce the risk of harm.

c. When psychologists become aware that research procedures have harmed a participant they take reasonable steps to minimize harm. (APA, 2002)

According to the APA, deception in research basically requires that the researcher (1) apply a cost/benefit analysis that explicitly considers the potential for harm created and/or exacerbated by the use of deception, (2) consider alternative methodologies, and (3) fully explain the nature of the deception at the conclusion of the study or explicitly justify withholding such information. In all cases, the safety and comfort of the participant should be of paramount concern.

GUIDELINES FOR THE CONSENT DOCUMENT

By definition, deceptive procedures eliminate the possibility of fully informed consent. As a consequence, the

APA code makes this explicit statement: "Psychologists never deceive research participants about significant aspects that would affect their willingness to participate" (2002, p. 807(b)). Although participants may not be fully informed, obviously they should be informed of as much as possible without threatening the ability of the researcher to test the true hypothesis of the study. Our recommendation is that the IRB should not approve a consent document that contains inaccurate information. The following specific guidelines apply:

- The consent document should *never* be used as part of the deception and thus should not include anything that is untrue.
- The consent document should reveal as much as possible to the participant regarding the procedures in the study.
- The consent document need not explain the details of the study if this will eliminate the capability of the study to inform the process under investigation. A useful guideline to keep in mind is that the experimenter–subject relationship is a real relationship "in which we have responsibility toward the subject as another human being whose dignity we must preserve."

REFERENCE

American Psychological Association. (2002). *Ethical principles of psychologists and code of conduct.* Available: http://www.apa.org/ethics/code/code.pdf.

Qualitative Social Science Research

DEAN R. GALLANT AND ROBERT AMDUR

Qualitative Research

- Informed consent is an important part of qualitative research. Much qualitative research is exploratory, and the areas of inquiry may not be apparent even to the research team at the time the study is initiated.
- Qualitative research should be designed to sustain the consent process throughout the course of a subject's participation.
- Qualitative researchers may encounter reportable situations—evidence of child or elder abuse or neglect, or the likely prospect of harm to self or others. Researchers who are likely to uncover reportable situations must be prepared for the possibility.
- If identifiers must be retained for long periods of time and if the research deals with sensitive topics, it may be appropriate to seek a certificate of confidentiality to protect against compelled disclosure—by federal, state, or local authorities.

Not all research fits the standard hypothesis-driven format. There is a long tradition of *qualitative research* by anthropologists, ethnographers, sociologists, survey researchers, psychologists, oral historians, and others whose observations are typically conducted outside the laboratory or clinical trial setting. The purpose of *qualitative* research is to develop hypotheses rather than to test and validate them. Methods include observation (including participant observation), questionnaires, surveys, interviewing, or review and analysis of existing data. Because of the potential range of activities involved, qualitative research can present special problems for IRBs, for investigators, and for the subjects themselves.

TYPES OF RISK IN QUALITATIVE RESEARCH

Breach of Confidentiality

Subjects routinely share the stories of their daily lives with friends and colleagues. But in many forms of qualitative social science research, an investigator collects information with the hope of publishing the results—not necessarily quoting the subjects' comments directly as a reporter might do, but often summarizing the cumulative knowledge gained from the research inquiry. If identities are poorly disguised, whether from others or from the participants themselves, then the subjects may risk embarrassment or more serious harm. Risks are not limited to published data; researchers should separate identifiers from sensitive data as soon as possible.

Violation of Privacy

Privacy refers to a state of being free from unsanctioned intrusion. Ordinarily, individuals have a right to privacy—that is, control over the extent, timing, and circumstances of sharing information about themselves with others. Violation of privacy contravenes the Belmont Report's principle of respect for persons.

Validation of Bad Behavior

Some research may unintentionally reinforce undesirable characteristics of research subjects. For example, an investigator studying recreational drug use among teens might need to develop a relationship of trust with the subjects, including being able to talk with them without criticizing their drug-taking behavior. A nonjudgmental relationship like this, with a senior university researcher, can have the unfortunate effect of persuading subjects that their behavior is acceptable to wise adults. In cases where study activities may encourage harmful behavior on the part of the subjects, it may be appropriate for the IRB to discuss its concerns with the investigator to help narrow the gap between strict scientific objectivity and responsible social values.

Risk of Harm to Others

Secondary research subjects are individuals who do not themselves participate in the study but about whom the investigator obtains information via interview or other hearsay means. In December 1999, the Office of Protection from Research Risks (now OHRP) cited failure to obtain informed consent from secondary subjects as a finding in a letter of suspension of IRB authority. Oral historians and genetics researchers, among others, reacted promptly, insisting that extension of this regulatory interpretation would effectively halt much of their research, because they could not possibly obtain informed consent from everybody about whom they indirectly received information. As of this writing, the question is unresolved, but OHRP has not rescinded its interpretation, so IRBs should at least consider whether special consideration should be given to secondary subjects in studies where primary informants provide information about others.

INFORMED CONSENT

Although the content may differ, informed consent is no less important in qualitative research than it is in hypothesis-driven studies. However, much qualitative research is exploratory, and the areas of inquiry may not be apparent even to the research team. For this reason it is often impossible to inform subjects of all of the potential research procedures and risks. Ideally, as in all forms of research, the consent process should be sustained throughout the course of a subject's participation. As the researcher refines the study, subjects should be reminded that participation is voluntary, and their understanding of the risks and benefits of participation should be refreshed.

REPORTABLE SITUATIONS

Some qualitative research deals with sensitive topics and looks deeply into subjects' daily lives. As a result, investigators may encounter reportable situations—evidence of child or elder abuse or neglect, or the likely prospect of harm to self or others. In most states, investigators have a legal obligation to report such situations to appropriate authorities. Researchers who are at all likely to uncover reportable situations must be prepared for the possibility. A strategy for alerting subjects to the need for reporting is essential; depending on the nature of the study and the subject population, this can involve mention of the reporting requirement as part of the informed consent process or a more ad hoc procedure when the likelihood of reportable situations is small.

CERTIFICATE OF CONFIDENTIALITY

Whether or not a researcher is studying behaviors likely to yield information about reportable situations, subjects' reputations, relationships, employability, or legal status may be threatened by disclosure of identifiable information. The law does not recognize any automatic privilege for social science or medical researchers, and thus research data are vulnerable to subpoena or other official inquiry. If identifiers must be retained and if the research deals with sensitive topics, it may be appropriate to seek a certificate of confidentiality to protect against compelled disclosure—by federal, state, or local authorities.

Certificates of confidentiality can be granted by the federal funding agency, upon application, and are also available to investigators without federal funding. These certificates do not prohibit the investigator from disclosing information (and, in some states, confidentiality certificate protections are overridden by mandated reporting requirements), but they do provide a measure of protection for research subjects that would not otherwise be available.

ORAL HISTORY
....

In 2003, an exchange between the Oral History Association (OHA) and OHRP led to the publication of a policy statement by the OHA indicating that most oral history interviewing projects are not subject to IRB review because they do not meet the regulatory definition of research involving human subjects. In particular, most oral history projects are not "designed to develop or contribute to generalizable knowledge" (45 CFR 46.102). The implications of this statement have energized debate in the oral history and IRB communities.

Subsequent correspondence and commentary by OHRP and others sought to clarify the situation. The issue is not simply whether a proposed project involves oral history interviews. IRBs should consider carefully whether a project collecting oral history data meets the federal definition of research involving human subjects.

REFERENCES
....

Protection of Human Subjects, 45 C. F. R. pt. 46 (2009).

Waiver or Alteration of Informed Consent or Documentation Thereof

MARIANNE M. ELLIOT AND ROBERT AMDUR

WAIVER OR ALTERATION OF INFORMED CONSENT

- The research involves no more than minimal risk to the subjects.
- The waiver or alteration will not adversely affect the rights and welfare of the subjects.
- The research could not practicably be carried out without the waiver or alteration.
- Whenever appropriate, the subjects will be provided with additional pertinent information after participation.

CIRCUMSTANCES WHEN AN IRB MAY WAIVE THE REQUIREMENT FOR DOCUMENTATION OF INFORMED CONSENT

- The only record linking the subject and the research would be the consent document, and the principal risk would be potential harm resulting from a breach of confidentiality. Each subject will be asked whether he or she wants documentation linking himself or herself with the research, and his or her wishes will govern.

continues

> **Waiver or Alteration of Informed Consent or Documentation Thereof** *continued*
> ....
> • The research presents no more than minimal risk of harm to subjects and involves no procedures for which written consent is normally required outside of the research context.

The purpose of this chapter is to explain the situations where federal regulations permit the IRB to approve research and waive the requirement for informed consent or the requirement for documentation of informed consent. A special case of the waiver of consent issue is the situation where research is conducted without consent in the setting of a medical emergency. There is an extensive list of requirements for IRB approval of research in the setting of a medical emergency that are described in federal regulations that were established specifically to deal with this controversial situation. The discussion in this chapter does not apply to the situation where research is conducted without consent in the setting of a medical emergency.

This chapter deals only with human research protection requirements under the Common Rule. Institutions and IRBs also must determine whether Health Insurance Portability and Accountability Act (HIPAA) requirements are met.

IRB WAIVER OR ALTERATION OF INFORMED CONSENT (45 CFR 46.116 [D])

An IRB may approve a consent procedure that does not include or which alters some or all of the elements of informed consent set forth in this section, or it may waive the requirement to obtain informed consent provided the IRB finds and documents the following:

- The research involves no more than minimal risk to the subjects.
- The waiver or alteration will not adversely affect the rights and welfare of the subjects.
- The research could not practicably be carried out without the waiver or alteration.
- Whenever appropriate, the subjects will be provided with additional pertinent information after participation.

Although the actual purpose of the research is to determine how mood may be related to body image, subjects are informed that the research is actually two separate research projects: one related to moods and how they may change and the other related to body image. This deception is part of the research design, and the student subjects are not fully informed about the purpose of the research.

In this example, the IRB may find that an alteration of informed consent is appropriate and that the criteria stated previously have been met based on the following:

1. **The research involves minimal risk**. The visual images are similar to those that the subjects might see in magazines about health and exercise or in movies. There are no provocative images. The questionnaires and scales are valid and reliable scales that are used in standard psychosocial testing.

Example 1
....

> The researcher plans to determine how mood and perception of one's body image may be related. Initially, subjects complete a series of written questionnaires and scales about their body image. After the subjects are presented with visual images intended to evoke a negative mood, the subjects are asked to complete the same questionnaires and scales. The effect of evoking a negative mood is evaluated.

2. **The rights and welfare of subjects are not adversely affected**. Subjects are informed about the actual procedures of the research, the lack of anticipated benefits, and the ability to discontinue participation at any time without penalty. Subjects are not informed that the research actually has only one purpose and that the data will be evaluated for that intent.

3. **The research could not practicably be carried out without the alteration in the informed consent process**. The research evaluates a feature of human behavior that is likely to be affected by the subjects' knowledge of the behavior that is being evaluated.

4. **In this research, it is appropriate to provide subjects with additional pertinent information after participation**. The researcher debriefs the subjects after their participation to explain the actual purpose of the research and why the research design was appropriate. The researcher also offers to be available for any questions subjects may have and provides information about appropriate services if subjects experience distress or anxiety about their participation in the research.

In this example, the IRB may find that a waiver of informed consent is appropriate and that the criteria stated previously have been met based on the following:

1. **The research involves minimal risk**. The review of medical records is for limited information, the information is not sensitive in nature, and the data are derived from clinically indicated procedures. The precautions taken to limit the record review to specified data and the double coding of the data further minimize the major risk, which is a breach of confidentiality.

Example 2
....

> *The researcher plans to determine whether blood chemistry values change in individuals undergoing clinically indicated abdominal surgery and if there is a correlation of changes with the increased incidence of complications after surgery. The researcher plans to review the medical records of all individuals who have undergone abdominal surgery in the past year and of those who will undergo surgery in the next year. From a preliminary estimate, there are about 1,000 abdominal surgeries performed per year at the hospital. The researcher will collect limited data for this for research. The types of data to be collected include such items as the diagnosis before surgery, the type of abdominal surgery, specific blood chemistry values before the surgery, the same specific blood chemistry values after the surgery, a description of problems after surgery, and perhaps the age ranges of the individuals. The researcher will double-code the data so that the link is known only to the researcher and no others, in the unlikely event the data must be verified for accuracy. The results of the research will not affect the clinical care of the individuals, because the information will not be examined until after subjects leave the hospital.*

2. **The rights and welfare of the individual would not be adversely affected**. The clinically indicated surgical procedure and the associated blood chemistry values were already completed, or would be completed, regardless of the research.

3. **The research could not be practicably carried out without the waiver**. Identifying and contacting the thousands of potential subjects, although not impossible, would not be feasible to get consent to review medical records.

4. **Providing subjects with additional information is not appropriate**. It would not be appropriate to provide these subjects with additional pertinent

information about the results of the research because the results would have no effect on the subjects.

IRB TO WAIVER OF THE DOCUMENTATION OF INFORMED CONSENT (45 CFR 46.117 [C])

Federal regulations describe the following two circumstances when an IRB may waive the requirement to obtain a signed consent form:

1. The only record linking the subject and the research would be the consent document, and the principal risk would be potential harm resulting from a breach of confidentiality. Each subject will be asked whether the subject wants documentation linking the subject with the research, and the subject's wishes will govern.

2. The research presents no more than minimal risk of harm to subjects and involves no procedures for which written consent is normally required outside of the research context.

In cases in which the documentation requirement is waived, the IRB may require the investigator to provide subjects with a written statement regarding the research.

Waiving the requirement for the investigator to obtain a signed consent form for some or all subjects means that the investigator obtains full and voluntary informed consent from every subject; however, the investigator does not require the subject to sign a consent document.

In this example, the IRB may waive the requirement to obtain a signed consent form because the research presents no more than minimal risk of harm to subjects. The questionnaire has no identifying information about the subject, and the purpose of the research is to evaluate the effectiveness of the program itself. Normally, there is no requirement for written consent for completion of written questionnaires outside the research context. By virtue of completing the questionnaire, subjects have consented to

Example 3
....

A researcher plans to evaluate the effectiveness of a smoking cessation program with women who are receiving prenatal care at the local health clinic. During prenatal visits, women who are already participating in the smoking cessation program will be asked to complete a written questionnaire about the program. The one-time written questionnaire includes questions about how well the women are complying with the program and how they feel about their progress. There is no identifying information about the woman on the questionnaire, and whether the woman completes the questionnaire has no effect on the care she may receive at the clinic.

participate in the research. In this case, the IRB may require the researcher to provide subjects with a written summary or an information sheet about the research.

In this example, the IRB determines that the only record linking the subject and the research would be the consent document. The principal risk would be potential harm resulting from a breach of confidentiality if the consent documents were disclosed, purposefully or inadvertently. To

Example 4
....

A researcher plans face-to-face interviews with university students who belong to a support group on campus for transgendered, gay, lesbian, and bisexual individuals. The purpose of the research is to evaluate the quality of healthcare services for these individuals. The researcher plans to recruit subjects through flyers and information distributed at support group meetings. Potential subjects will contact the researcher directly. The researcher plans to conduct two face-to-face interviews 6 months apart. The interviews will be audiotaped, and the researcher will ask subjects to use a pseudonym during the interviews. Also, each subject will be assigned a coded number on the audiotape.

minimize the potential harm to subjects, the IRB may permit the informed consent process to be conducted verbally and have the researcher document, perhaps in a research note, the circumstances of the consent process. The IRB may then request that the researcher ask subjects whether they want documentation linking them with the research, and each subject's wishes will be honored.

The IRB may also require the researcher to provide each subject with a written summary or information sheet about the research. However, in this example, even having an information sheet about the research could be potentially harmful to subjects who may already suffer from social stigma, embarrassment, or ostracism. The IRB may suggest providing subjects with a card with only the name and phone number of the researcher in the event they have any questions or concerns.

It may be useful for the IRB to require that the investigator inform each subject about the temporal aspects of the risks associated with a signed consent document as the only link between the subject and the research. Subjects, as students or activists, might feel that the immediate potential harm from having a document with their signature confirming their participation in the research is minimal and a potential breach of confidentiality is not relevant. In contrast, the same subjects may find the harm caused by an inadvertent breach of confidentiality perhaps 5–10 years later during a job interview to be greater.

Exculpatory Language in the Consent Document

CHAPTER 3-10

MICHELE RUSSELL-EINHORN, THOMAS PUGLISI, AND ROBERT AMDUR

Exculpatory Language in the Consent Document

The IRB should consider *exculpatory language* to be any language through which the subject or the representative is made to waive or appear to waive *any* of the subject's legal rights. An informed consent document that includes words like, *I authorize*; *I understand*; *I agree*; or *I have been advised* should be viewed as red flags raising the specter of exculpatory language.

- The following statements are examples of exculpatory language:
    1. I agree that the medical center will not pay me for any injuries that I might sustain as a result of participating in this research.
    2. I understand that the institution will not share with me any profits received from the sale or commercialization of any cells developed in this research.
    3. I understand that I will not sue the sponsor or the investigator for any negligence.
    4. Subjects agree to hold harmless all institutions, investigators, or sponsors affiliated with or in any way a part of this research protocol.

Investigators are frequently admonished by their IRBs to refrain from using exculpatory language in their informed consent documents (and, just as importantly, throughout the consent process). Almost as frequently, this admonishment comes with little or no explanation of what constitutes exculpatory language. Indeed, many IRBs seem confused about where to draw the line in determining whether a proposed statement is exculpatory. Here is what federal regulations say about exculpatory language in the consent process:

> No informed consent, whether oral or written, may include any exculpatory language through which the subject is made to waive or appear to waive any of the subject's legal rights, or releases or appears to release the investigator, the sponsor, the institution, or its agents from liability for negligence. (45 CFR 46.116)

THE NARROW (BUT INCORRECT) INTERPRETATION

A narrow interpretation of the regulatory language would limit the prohibition to specific situations where one can point to a law that provides or appears to provide subjects with specific rights. Thus, a statement in an informed consent document stating that subjects release the investigator from any liability for negligence would clearly be a waiver of a subject's right to sue someone for negligent conduct. Those who argue in favor of the narrow interpretation point out that in common usage (as verified by any current dictionary), the word *exculpatory* relates to lack of guilt. This is also the case relative to its usage in law. According to *Black's Law Dictionary*, the word involves clearing "from alleged fault or guilt" or releasing "from liability" for "wrongful acts."

THE BROAD (CORRECT) INTERPRETATION

These arguments notwithstanding, the federal agencies that regulate research have a long history of applying a much broader interpretation of the exculpatory language prohibition. A careful reading of the regulatory language reveals that, in this context, the meaning of the phrase *exculpatory language* is expanded to include any language "through which the subject or the representative is made to waive or appear to waive any of the subject's legal rights" (45 CFR 46.116). Thus any language waiving or appearing to waive any legal right (regardless of the nature of that right) is prohibited. There is also an absence of guidance as to what constitutes a legal right, because this may vary from state to state.

PRACTICAL APPLICATIONS

In a practical sense, exculpatory statements tend to be statements in which a subject in a research protocol is asked to agree to or accept something, usually something unfavorable to the subject. A statement that sets forth simple facts, on the other hand, is usually not exculpatory.

Examples of Language That Is *Not Exculpatory*

In the following examples, the institution simply sets forth the facts describing the institution's intent and policy. These statements would not be exculpatory under the regulations.

1. The University Medical School has no policy or plan to pay for any injuries you might receive as a result of participating in this research protocol.

2. Tissue obtained from you in this research may be used to establish a cell line that could be patented and licensed. There are no plans to provide financial compensation to you should this occur.

Examples of Exculpatory Language

1. I agree that the medical center will not pay me for any injuries that I might sustain as a result of participating in this research.

2. I understand that the institution will not share with me any profits received from the sale or commercialization of any cells developed in this research.

3. I understand that I will not sue the sponsor or the investigator for any negligence.

4. Subjects agree to hold harmless all institutions, investigators, or sponsors affiliated with or in any way a part of this research protocol.

Again, a good rule of thumb is to state simply the factual situation and avoid any statement that requires the agreement or concurrence of the subject.

REFERENCES

Protection of Human Subjects, 45 C. F. R. pt. 46 (2009).

When Are Research Risks Reasonable in Relation to Anticipated Benefits?

CHARLES WEIJER AND PAUL B. MILLER

Component Analysis

- Component analysis is built on the recognition that clinical research often contains a mixture of therapeutic and nontherapeutic procedures.
- Research risks are reasonable in relation to anticipated benefits when the IRB determines that the moral standards for both therapeutic and nontherapeutic procedures are fulfilled.

The question "when are research risks reasonable in relationship to anticipated benefits?" is at the very heart of pressing disputes in the ethics of clinical research. Institutional review boards (IRBs) are criticized for inconsistent decision making, a phenomenon that may be traced in part to reliance on the vagaries of intuition to interpret federal regulation on acceptable risks and potential benefits (Shah, Whittle, Wilfond, Gensler, & Wendler, 2004). Furthermore, the problem of acceptability of risks and potential benefits in research runs through a number of contemporary controversies, including the ethics of research involving placebo controls (Emanuel & Miller, 2001), developing countries (Angell, 1997), incapable adults

(Karlawish, 2003), and emergency rooms (Valenzuela & Copass, 2001). If IRBs are to be given clear guidance, and if pressing ethical questions are to be addressed in a principled way, then a systematic approach to the ethics of risk in research is required.

A systematic approach to the ethical analysis of risks and potential benefits in research called "component analysis" has recently been developed (Weijer, 2000). Component analysis is built on the recognition that clinical research often contains a mixture of therapeutic and nontherapeutic procedures and that separate moral standards are required for each. (See Figure 3-11.1.)

COMPONENT ANALYSIS PROVIDES
CLEAR CRITERIA FOR IRBS

The Common Rule instructs IRBs to ensure that "risks to subjects are minimized" and "risks to subjects are reasonable in relation to anticipated benefits, if any, to subjects, and the importance of the knowledge that may be reasonably expected to result" (45 CFR 46.111[a][1,2]). Unembellished imperatives often provoke more questions than they answer. Which risks to subjects must be minimized? To what extent must they be minimized? Which risks and which potential benefits are to be considered in the reasonableness determinations? By what measure does one determine that risks are reasonable in relationship to benefits to subjects? By what measure does one determine that risks are reasonable in relation to the knowledge that may result? In the absence of careful explication of these regulatory requirements, it is difficult to see how IRBs can effectively fulfill their mandate of protecting research subjects (U.S. National Bioethics Advisory Commission, 2000).

Component analysis builds on the recognition that clinical trials often contain a mixture of interventions administered with differing purposes. Drug, surgical, and behavioral interventions are administered with therapeutic warrant; that is, they are administered on the basis of evidence sufficient to justify the belief that they may benefit research subjects. Other interventions, such as venipuncture for pharmacokinetic drug levels, additional imaging procedures, or questionnaires not used in clinical practice, are given without therapeutic warrant. They are administered solely for the purpose of answering the scientific question. Because this distinction is morally relevant, IRBs must apply separate moral standards to their assessment of therapeutic and nontherapeutic procedures.

Therapeutic procedures must meet the ethical standard of clinical equipoise (Freedman, 1987). Clinical equipoise is a research-friendly response to this question: "When may a physician offer enrollment in a clinical trial to his or her patient?" It provides that he or she may do so when the therapeutic procedures in a clinical trial are consistent with competent medical care. More formally, clinical equipoise requires that at the outset of a trial there exists a state of honest, professional disagreement in the community of expert practitioners as to the preferred treatment. Procedurally, the IRB does not make this determination by surveying practitioners. Rather, it scrutinizes the study justification, reviews relevant literature, and when required, consults with independent clinical experts. Clinical equipoise is satisfied if the IRB concludes that the evidence supporting the various therapeutic procedures is sufficient that, if it were widely known, expert clinicians would disagree as to the preferred treatment.

Nontherapeutic procedures do not offer the prospect of direct benefit to research subjects. When assessing risks associated with nontherapeutic procedures (nontherapeutic risks), the IRB must determine that two separate ethical standards are met. The IRB must determine that nontherapeutic risks are, first, minimized consistent with sound scientific design and, second, reasonable in relationship to the knowledge that may be gained from the study. Procedurally, the IRB ensures that nontherapeutic risks are minimized by, where feasible, requiring the substitution of "procedures already being performed on the subjects for diagnostic and treatment purposes" (45 CFR 46.111[a][1][ii]).

When research involves a vulnerable population, such as pregnant women, prisoners, or children, additional

Figure 3-11.1 Component analysis of risks and potential benefits in research

....

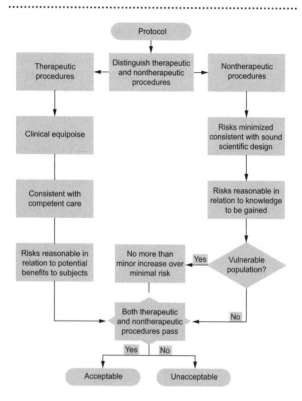

protection may be required. A threshold may be invoked limiting the nontherapeutic risks to which vulnerable subjects may be exposed. For children, nontherapeutic risks are limited to the standard of a minor increase over minimal risk. In other words, a minor increase over the risks "ordinarily encountered in daily life" (45 CFR 46.406[a], 46.102[i]). Procedurally, to determine whether the risks of nontherapeutic procedures fulfill this criterion, the IRB reasons by analogy (Freedman, Fuks, & Weijer, 1993). It asks whether risks posed by nontherapeutic procedures are the same as those ordinarily encountered in daily life or are sufficiently similar to these risks (45 CFR 46.102[i]). Whether the referent for minimal risk ought to be the daily lives of healthy or sick children remains controversial (Kopelman, 2000; Miller & Weijer, 2000).

Research risks are reasonable in relationship to anticipated benefits when the IRB determines that the moral standards for both therapeutic and nontherapeutic procedures are fulfilled.

ACKNOWLEDGMENTS

The authors are grateful to C. Heilig at the Centers for Disease Control and Prevention for preparing Figure 3-11.1. This work was supported by a Canadian Institutes of Health Research Investigator Award and Operating Grant (C.W.) and a doctoral fellowship from the Social Sciences and Humanities Research Council of Canada (P.B.M.).

REFERENCES

Angell, M. (1997). The ethics of clinical research in the third world. *New England Journal of Medicine, 337*, 847–849.

Emanuel, E. J., & Miller F. G. (2001). The ethics of placebo-controlled trials: A middle ground. *New England Journal of Medicine, 345*, 915–919.

Freedman, B. (1987). Equipoise and the ethics of clinical research. *New England Journal of Medicine, 317*, 141–145.

Freedman, B., Fuks, A., & Weijer, C. (1993). In loco parentis: minimal risk as an ethical threshold for research upon children. *Hastings Center Report, 23*(2), 13–19.

Karlawish, J. H. (2003). Research involving cognitively impaired adults. *New England Journal of Medicine, 348*, 1389–1392.

Kopelman, L. M. (2000). Children as research subjects: A dilemma. *The Journal of Medicine and Philosophy, 25*, 745–764.

Miller, P. B. & Weijer, C. (2000). Moral solutions in assessing research risk. *IRB, 22*, 6–10.

Protection of Human Subjects, 45 C. F. R. pt. 46 (2009).

Shah, S., Whittle, A., Wilfond, B., Gensler., G., & Wendler, D. (2004). How do IRBs apply the federal risk and benefit standards for pediatric research? *JAMA, 291*, 476–482.

U.S. National Bioethics Advisory Commission. (2000). *Ethical and policy issues in research involving human participants.* Bethesda, MD: U.S. National Bioethics Advisory Commission, p. 13.

Valenzuela, T. D., & Copass, M. K. (2001). Clinical research on out-of-hospital emergency care. *New England Journal of Medicine, 345,* 689–690.

Weijer, C. J. (2000). The ethical analysis of risk. *Journal of Law, Medicine & Ethics, 28,* 344–361.

Research Involving Children

ROBERT NELSON AND ROBERT AMDUR

Research Involving Children

Federal regulations permit the IRB to approve research involving children *only* if the research interventions or procedures fall into one of the following three categories:

1. Research involving no greater than minimal risk to children.

2. Research involving an intervention or procedure presenting more than minimal risk to children that offers the prospect of direct benefit or may contribute to the well-being of the individual child. In addition, the risks must be justified by the anticipated benefit to the subjects, and the relation of the anticipated benefit to the risk must be at least as favorable as that presented by available alternative approaches.

3. Research involving an intervention or procedure that presents only a minor increase over minimal risk, yet does not offer any prospect of direct benefit or contribute to the well-being of the child. In addition, the intervention or procedure must present experiences to the subjects that are similar with their actual or expected situations, and likely yield generalizable knowledge of vital importance for understanding or ameliorating the child's disorder or condition.

THE ADDITIONAL SAFEGUARDS
FOR CHILDREN IN RESEARCH

All of the ethical standards and regulatory requirements that apply to adults are required for the conduct of research involving children. In addition, 45 CFR 46 Subpart D of the HHS regulations (and corresponding sections of 21 CFR 50 for FDA-regulated research) contain additional safeguards that the IRB must consider for research involving children. These safeguards follow two general approaches, based on the presence or absence of the prospect of direct benefit. First, when an intervention or procedure does not offer the prospect of direct benefit, the appropriate level of risk exposure is limited to either minimal risk (for any child) or a minor increase over minimal risk (for a child with the condition being studied). This restriction in allowable risk exposure corresponds to two categories of research involving children that allow for exposure to either minimal risk or a minor increase over minimal risk. Second, when an intervention and/or procedure offers the prospect of direct benefit, the justification for acceptable risk exposure is limited to conditions approximating research equipoise. Thus the regulations permit the IRB to approve research involving children *only* if it falls into one of the following categories:

- **Research presenting no greater than minimal risk to children**. The IRB determines that the level of risk is no greater than minimal, regardless of whether the research offers the prospect of direct benefit to the child. The level of risk that a child may be exposed to by interventions and/or procedures that do not offer the prospect of direct benefit is restricted to the level of risk that a child may be exposed to in the course of a child's everyday life. An intervention and/or procedure that offers the prospect of direct benefit yet presents only minimal risk is also approvable under this category.

- **Research involving an intervention or procedure presenting more than minimal risk to children that offers the prospect of direct benefit or may contribute to the well-being of the individual child**. The IRB may approve an intervention or procedure that offers the prospect of direct benefit to the individual child (or a monitoring procedure that is likely to contribute to the subject's well-being), and presents greater than minimal risk only if (1) the risk is justified by the anticipated benefit to the subjects and (2) the relation of the anticipated benefit to the risk is at least as favorable to the subjects as that presented by available alternative approaches. In effect, each arm of a study must have an appropriate risk/benefit balance, and the comparative therapeutic merits of each arm of a clinical trial should be balanced. The alternatives that must be considered include any available alternatives outside of the research study. The general principle is that a child should not be disadvantaged by entering a research study. A parent's decision to enroll a child in research should be similar to a decision to permit exposure to the risks and benefits of any nonresearch alternative.

- **Research involving an intervention or procedure that presents only a minor increase over minimal risk, yet does not offer any prospect of direct benefit or contribute to the well-being of the child**. The limited conditions under which such research can be approved by an IRB include the following: (1) the risk represents only a minor increase over minimal risk; (2) the intervention or procedure presents experiences to subjects that are reasonably commensurate with those inherent in their actual or expected medical, dental, psychological, social, or educational situations; or (3) the intervention or procedure is likely to yield generalizable knowledge about the subject's disorder or condition, which is of vital importance for the understanding or amelioration of the subject's disorder or condition.

All three categories require that adequate provisions are made for soliciting assent of the children and permission of their parents or guardians.

If an IRB cannot fit the research into one of these three categories, it must disapprove the research or refer it to a special review panel reporting to either the secretary of the HHS or the FDA commissioner. However, before a research project can be referred to a federal panel, the local IRB must determine that "the research presents a reasonable opportunity to further the understanding, prevention, or alleviation of a serious problem affecting the health or welfare of children" (45 CFR 46.407(a)).

MINIMAL RISK AND A MINOR INCREASE OVER MINIMAL RISK

Guidelines under discussion at the federal level interpret minimal risk for research involving children to be that level of risk associated with the daily activities of a normal, healthy, average child. Risks include all harms, discomforts, indignities, embarrassments, and potential breaches of privacy and confidentiality associated with the research. Whether or not an intervention or procedure qualifies as minimal risk is not simply a statistical judgment, nor does it merely reflect that the risks associated with a procedure have been minimized. Conceptually, the minimal-risk standard defines a permissible level of risk in research as the socially (or normatively) allowable risks that parents generally permit their children to be exposed to in nonresearch situations.

Healthy children experience differing levels of risk in their daily lives. Indexing minimal risk to the socially (or normatively) allowable risks to which normal, average, healthy children are exposed routinely accounts for the differing risks experienced by children of different ages. However, the fact that some children may be exposed to differing levels of risk in the course of their daily lives may not justify greater risk exposure. If certain groups of children are routinely exposed to greater risks as part of their daily lives because of the circumstances in which they live, this level of increased risk ought *not* be interpreted as minimal risk just because it is part of the common experience of these otherwise healthy children. The phrase, *ordinarily encountered in the daily life or during the performance of routine physical or psychological examinations or tests*, is interpreted to mean an equivalence of risk rather than the procedure being one that is actually performed routinely. Thus a test or procedure that entails minimal risk is one for which the probability and magnitude of risk associated with the test or procedure is equivalent to and no greater than the risk of events ordinarily encountered in the daily life of a normal, healthy, average child, or the socially (or normatively) allowable risks parents permit their normal, healthy, average children to be exposed to in their ordinary lives.

A minor increase over minimal risk refers to those risks that are slightly more than minimal and pose no significant threat to the child's health or well-being. While minimal risk is indexed to the risks encountered in the daily lives of normal, healthy, average children, the permissible level of risk associated with a minor increase over minimal should only be slightly more than that level and also commensurate with the risks of interventions or procedures having been experienced or expected to be experienced in the lives of children with a specific disorder or condition. Although some children may experience invasive procedures with considerable risk and discomfort during the care and treatment of a disease, this does not justify risks greater than a minor increase over minimal in a research study that provides no prospect of direct benefit to the individual subjects. In addition, this level of risk must be necessary in order to yield generalizable knowledge of vital importance for the understanding of the participants' disorder or condition.

DISORDER AND/OR CONDITION

The phrase *disorder and/or condition* refers to a characteristic of the group of potential research subjects and implies that this characteristic can be understood more broadly than simply a specific disease or diagnostic category. Generally, the concept of disorder or condition relates to a specific characteristic that describes a group of children, such as a physical or social condition affecting children, or the risk of certain children developing a disease in the future based on diagnostic testing or physical examination. For example, prematurity, infancy, adolescence, poverty, living in a compromised physical environment, institutionalization, or having a genetic predisposition to future illness may be considered a disorder or condition in the context of an appropriate research protocol that, under the appropriate circumstances, warrants permissible research that presents levels of risk that are a minor increase over minimal levels without the prospect of direct benefit.

Approving Research Without Parental Permission

Federal regulations permit the IRB to approve research without the permission of a parent "if the IRB determines that a research protocol is designed for conditions or for a subject population for which ... permission is not a reasonable requirement to protect the subjects (for example, neglected or abused children), provided an appropriate mechanism for protecting the children who will participate as subjects in the research is substituted, and provided further that the waiver is not inconsistent with federal, state, or local law" (45 CFR 46.408(c)). For example, many pediatric IRBs will waive the requirement for parental permission for research using adolescent subjects that involves medical procedures and treatment that the adolescent can consent to without parental knowledge, such as use of contraceptives, treatment of sexually transmitted disease, treatment of alcohol and drug abuse, and so forth. However, the FDA does not allow the waiver of parental permission for research involving an FDA-regulated product.

CHILD ASSENT

Assent is defined as "a child's affirmative agreement to participate in research" (45 CFR 46.402(b)). A child's passive resignation to submit to an intervention or procedure must not be considered assent. The federal regulations do not specify any of the elements of informed assent and do not indicate an age at which assent ought to be possible. Assent should be tailored to the level of comprehension of the child.

An IRB is granted wide discretion in determining whether a child is capable of assenting and can waive the requirement for child assent under the following circumstances: if a child is not capable of assent; if the research offers a prospect of direct benefit not available outside of the research (thus falling under the scope of parental authority in overriding a child's desires); or given the same conditions under which parental permission can be waived. An IRB is granted wide discretion in determining whether and how a child's assent is documented.

REFERENCE

Protection of Human Subjects, 45 C. F. R. pt. 46 (2009).

Regulatory Issues of Research Involving Prisoners

CHRISTOPHER J. KRATOCHVIL,
ERNEST D. PRENTICE, BRUCE G. GORDON,
AND GAIL D. KOTULAK

Research Involving Prisoners

In addition to the requirements for IRB approval that apply to all research, federal regulations require additional protections that are required for the IRB to approve research that involves prisoners, including the following:

- Any potential benefits from research participation are not coercive in the limited-choice environment of the prison.
- The risks involved in the research are commensurate with risks that would be accepted by nonprisoner volunteers.
- The procedures for the selection of subjects within the prison are fair to all prisoners and immune from arbitrary intervention by prison authorities or prisoners.
- Participation in the research will have no effect on parole determinations.

Prisoners are considered a vulnerable subject population in need of additional protections, defined as follows in federal regulations:

> "Prisoner" means any individual involuntarily confined or detained in a penal institution. The term is intended to encompass individuals sentenced to such an institution under a criminal or civil statute as well as individuals detained in other facilities by virtue of statutes or commitment procedures which provide alternatives to criminal prosecution or incarceration in a penal institution, and individuals detained pending arraignment, trial, or sentencing.

One of the difficulties in the use of Subpart C of the federal regulations (45 CFR 46) lies within the definition of *prisoner.* Many of the current alternatives to incarceration, such as house arrest with electronic monitoring, were not in existence at the time of the writing of Subpart C. Additionally, while many others may not meet the definition of a prisoner per se (such as parolees or probationers, persons court-ordered to attend nonresidential treatment programs in the community, and those adjudicated to reside in halfway houses), all have impingements on their freedom and the potential for coercion. For these vulnerable subjects who may not be protected under Subpart C, they should be afforded additional protections under Subpart A in the charge to the IRB to "be particularly cognizant of the special problems of research involving vulnerable populations …" (45 CFR 46.111(a) (3)).

COMPOSITION OF THE IRB

According to federal regulations at 45 CFR 46.304(a)(b), the IRB reviewing prisoner research must be specially constituted. The board must include at least one member who is a prisoner or a prisoner representative with the appropriate background and experience to serve in that capacity. The IRB must be so constituted for all reviews of research involving prisoners, including initial review, continuing review, protocol amendments, and review of adverse events. If a human subject participating in an IRB-approved protocol becomes a prisoner after the research has begun, the protocol and consent document would need to be reviewed by the IRB again, with a prisoner representative present. Unless the IRB reapproves the research for inclusion of the prisoner(s), the newly incarcerated individual must be withdrawn from the study. OHRP has provided guidance that allows one important exception, however. "In special circumstances in which the principal investigator asserts that it is in the best interests of the subject to remain in the research study while incarcerated, the IRB Chairman may determine that the subject may continue to participate in the research until the requirements of Subpart C are satisfied" (OHRP, 2003).

IRB APPROVAL CRITERIA FOR PRISONER RESEARCH

As with all other types of research, prisoner research must comply with the requirements of the general ethical codes and regulations that apply to research that does not involve prisoners. These requirements are that the risks to subjects must be minimized; risks to subjects are reasonable in relation to anticipated benefits; the selection of subjects is equitable; informed consent is obtained and appropriately documented; the research plan makes adequate provision for monitoring the data collected to ensure the safety of subjects; and there are adequate provisions to protect the privacy of subjects and to maintain the confidentiality of data.

Federal regulations require the following additional protections for prisoners by setting further conditions that must all be satisfied before the IRB can approve the study:

1. The research under review represents one of the categories of research permissible under 45 CFR 46.306(a)(2).

2. Any possible advantages accruing to the prisoner through his or her participation in the research,

when compared to the general living conditions, medical care, quality of food, amenities and opportunity for earnings in the prison, are not of such a magnitude that his or her ability to weigh the risks of the research against the value of such advantages in the limited choice environment of the prison is impaired.

3. The risks involved in the research are commensurate with risks that would be accepted by nonprisoner volunteers.

4. The procedures for the selection of subjects within the prison are fair to all prisoners and immune from arbitrary intervention by prison authorities or prisoners. Unless the principal investigator provides to the board justification in writing for following some other procedures, control subjects must be selected randomly from the group of available prisoners who meet the characteristics needed for that particular research project.

5. The information is presented in language that is understandable to the subject population.

6. Adequate assurance exists that parole boards will not take into account a prisoner's participation in the research in making decisions regarding parole, and each prisoner is clearly informed in advance that participation in the research will have no effect on his or her parole.

7. If the board finds that there may be a need for follow-up examination or care of participants after the end of their participation, adequate provision has been made for such examination or care, taking into account the varying lengths of individual prisoners' sentences, and for informing participants of this fact.

It should be noted that the last requirement is unclear in terms of how and to what extent the investigator, institution, or sponsor is responsible for providing care to both prisoners and parolees after their participation in research. Interpretation of this requirement is particularly problematic in clinical research on life-threatening illnesses such as cancer or AIDS where the patient is likely to need continued treatment, perhaps for a prolonged period and at considerable expense.

Research involving prisoners may not be exempted under Section 46.101(b). In addition, OHRP recommends that all prisoner research, even if technically expeditable under Section 46.110, should be reviewed by the full IRB with a prisoner or prisoner representative present at a convened meeting.

PROTECTION AT THE EXPENSE OF JUSTICE

The seven additional protections described previously are obviously designed to protect the rights and welfare of prisoners who participate in research. It is ironic, however, that these additional requirements also restrict the right of prisoners to participate in research. The result may be a paternalistic set of regulations that limit a prisoner's autonomy to decide to participate in and benefit from taking part in research. The Belmont principle of justice requires that both the benefits and burdens of research be distributed fairly. Also, by denying prisoners the ability to make a decision as to whether they want to participate in research, the Belmont principle of respect for persons may be violated. It is important for the IRB to consider these trade-offs when evaluating research that involves prisoners.

REFERENCE

Protection of Human Subjects, 45 C. F. R. pt. 46 (2009).

Placebo-Controlled Trials

ROBERT AMDUR

Evaluating the Ethics of a Placebo-Controlled Trial

Decision points in the algorithm for evaluating the ethics of a placebo-controlled trial are as follows:

- Is placebo used in place of, or in addition to, standard therapy?
- Is standard therapy considered to be effective?
- Is the toxicity of standard therapy such that patients routinely refuse treatment?
- Could the use of a placebo in place of standard therapy cause severe suffering or irreversible harm?
- Is it possible to estimate the placebo response rate in this study with a reasonable degree of accuracy?
- Evaluate the credibility of altruism using the reasonable-person standard. Could this trial benefit future patients to the point that a reasonable person with an average degree of altruism and risk aversiveness would consent to being randomized in this trial?

The ethics of using a placebo in medical research is controversial. At one end of the spectrum is the argument that the use of a placebo is unethical because alternate study designs would produce results that are of similar value to society with less risk to individual research participants. The counterargument is that placebo treatment is often ethically sound to protect society from the harm that would result from the widespread use of ineffective medical treatments. Figure 3-14.1 shows a decision algorithm that will help IRB members evaluate the ethics of a clinical research trial that involves concomitant placebo control.

THE USE OF PLACEBO IN PLACE OF STANDARD THERAPY

The first step in evaluating the ethics of a placebo-controlled trial is to decide if a placebo is being used in place of standard therapy. Standard therapy may be a type of active treatment, supportive care, or no treatment.

The potential problem with placebo therapy is that it exposes patients to a treatment that has no specific activity for their disease. When an available therapy is considered to be beneficial, the use of a placebo instead of accepted therapy may be unethical. However, there is no ethical problem when a placebo is being used in addition to standard therapy, as is done in add-on and sequential treatment study designs.

The Efficacy of Standard Therapy

The second decision point is to determine if standard therapy is considered to be effective. With medical conditions where there are no good treatment options, there may be legitimate controversy about the value of standard therapy.

When standard therapy does not meaningfully improve length or quality of life, it is ethical to enroll informed subjects in research that uses a placebo in place of standard treatment. However, when local physicians consider standard therapy to be effective in the study population, the IRB must evaluate additional issues to determine if it is ethical to use a placebo in place of standard therapy.

THE TOXICITY OF STANDARD TREATMENT

When evaluating the potential benefit of a medical treatment, it is important to consider both efficacy and toxicity. If the toxicity of standard treatment is such that patients routinely refuse this therapy or local physicians

Figure 3-14.1 *Source:* Amdur, R., & Biddle, C. J. (2001). An algorithm for evaluating the ethics of a placebo-controlled trial. *International Journal of Cancer, 96*(5), 261–269.

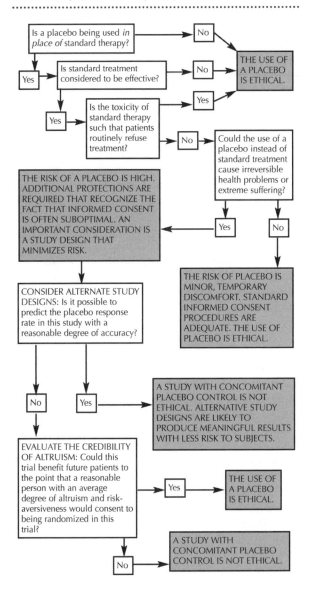

do not recommend the therapy, then it is ethical to conduct research that treats informed subjects with placebo in place of standard therapy, even when standard therapy is proven to have activity for their condition.

Temporary Discomfort Versus Irreversible Harm

Much of the recent literature on ethical requirements for the use of placebos has emphasized the importance of making a distinction between temporary discomfort and irreversible harm. The basic concept is that the study should take extra steps to be sure that subjects understand the risks and alternatives when they are considering participation in a study where the risk of placebo treatment is high.

When the risk of research participation is high, any imperfection in the consent process has a major effect on research ethics. When the use of placebo carries a risk of irreversible and serious harm, the ethics of research will hinge on the ability of alternate study designs to provide valuable information on the study question with less risk to research subjects.

Considering Alternative Study Designs

A fundamental ethical standard is that research should be designed so that the risks to subjects are minimized and reasonable in relation to anticipated benefits. A major element of the placebo controversy is debate over the implications of using alternative study designs to evaluate the efficacy of new medical treatments.

As a society, we want to design clinical trials to minimize the chance of a false-positive result. The scientific quality of a clinical trial refers to the aspects of the study that influence the persuasiveness of research results. The relationship between study quality and the use of concomitant placebo control is a complex and controversial topic. The main issue is the value of a positive result in a trial with placebo versus active control. An explanation of this topic is beyond the scope of this handbook but a major factor is if it is possible to estimate the placebo response rate with a reasonable degree of accuracy.

EVALUATING THE CREDIBILITY OF ALTRUISM USING THE REASONABLE-PERSON STANDARD

In a medical research study where the use of placebo increases the risk of major suffering or irreversible harm, the only way to justify the use of placebo is to argue that it is ethical to increase risk to current subjects to produce information that may benefit people in the future. A major problem with this argument is that the major guidelines related to research ethics stress the importance of not sacrificing the individual for the sake of society. Clearly there are situations where the trade-off between individual welfare and societal benefit is acceptable, but each person who is asked to be a research subject should be permitted to decide what is acceptable and unacceptable based on personal values.

There is no question that altruism may be an acceptable reason for a person to participate in research, regardless of the potential for increased risk. However, to accept the altruism argument, one must assume full and voluntary informed consent. When considering this argument, it is important to understand that an extensive body of literature now exists supporting the view that, in many medical situations, it is difficult for a subject to give the level of informed consent that is a requirement for ethical research. In studies on this subject, research subjects signed a valid consent document but did not understand the essential elements of informed consent for the study that they were going to participate in. There is no definitive formula for determining when a trade-off between the welfare of individual subjects and future patients is acceptable. A bioethicist named Baruch Brody suggests a reasonable-person standard for evaluating the ethics of clinical trials. In the context of the placebo discussion, the reasonable-person standard says that a randomized, placebo-controlled trial is justified only if both of these conditions exist:

1. the subjects have validly consented to being randomized, and

2. a reasonable person of an average degree of altruism and risk-aversiveness might consent to being randomized.

Phase 1 Oncology Trials

Matthew Miller and Robert Amdur

Phase 1 Oncology Trials

Phase 1 oncology trials are designed to produce significant toxicity with no planned direct benefit to research subjects.

- Therapeutic misconception often explains why people participate in Phase 1 oncology trials—meaning that they falsely believe that the study is designed to help them.
- Require standardized wording in the consent document as follows:
  Purpose: The purpose of this study is to find the highest dose of ____ that people can tolerate without getting extremely ill.
  Risks: In this study, the dose of _____ will be increased until people get extremely sick. It is impossible to predict the side effects that you will experience.
  Benefits: This study is not being done to treat your cancer. Phase 1 studies are neither designed nor expected to provide benefits to subjects. The main purpose of a Phase 1 study is to determine the highest tolerated dose of a new drug. We hope to gather information that may help people in the future.

A fundamental tension in human experimentation on patients arises from the inherent conflict between the goals of science and those of clinical care. Phase 1 cancer trials embody this conflict in perhaps its purest and most intensified form because the subjects in these trials are terminally ill patients and the scientific goal is to effect toxicity—not cure, remission, or palliation. This presents special challenges to IRB review, especially in light of empirical evidence that patients overwhelmingly enroll in these trials seeking physical benefit. The bioethicist Benjamin Freedman summarized the fundamental issue:

> A Phase 1 study of drug X is often said to be a study of X's safety and efficacy. Calling a toxicity study a study of safety seems harmless, and perhaps even reflects a laudably optimistic view of the world. Calling it a study of efficacy is, however, simply false; although to be sure, were there no hope of this drug's working it would not be tested. (Freedman)

BACKGROUND

In the course of developing new anticancer compounds, agents that have demonstrated promise in cell culture and animal models must at some time be tested in human subjects. In these initial or *Phase 1* human trials, compounds are administered to terminally ill cancer patients in an attempt to estimate the highest dose human beings can tolerate. Evaluating a drug's anticancer effect in human cancers, a primary objective of subsequent Phase 2 and Phase 3 trials, is not a defined goal in Phase 1 studies.

Phase 1 dose-toxicity information is usually gathered by administering increasing doses of a new drug (or of novel combinations of known agents) to successive cohorts of three to six patients. Once serious but reversible toxic effects are produced in a fixed proportion of patients (often one-third of the patients in the highest-dose cohort), the trial ends. Because most responses occur at 80–120% of the maximum tolerated dose, subjects enrolled in the earliest cohorts have the least risk of severe toxicity but also the least likelihood of a clinical response. Thus the predominant cohort-specific dose escalation schemes are at odds with what patients generally assume about the primacy of their interests—for example, that each patient will receive a dose that attempts to maximize the chance for anticancer effect.

THERAPEUTIC MISCONCEPTIONS OF SUBJECTS

There is now a large body of evidence that recognizes the process of therapeutic misconception—a misunderstanding whereby patients do not fully recognize the way that science sometimes deprives them of care chosen solely out of concern for their well-being. The chance of meaningful clinical benefit from participating in a Phase 1 cancer trial is almost zero, and the study is designed to push the dose of the study drug until toxicity is unacceptable. But most of the participants in Phase 1 cancer trials say that they are enrolling in these trials because they think that the main purpose of the trial is to make them better.

RECOMMENDATIONS FOR THE IRB

1. Determine if the study agent is being evaluated simultaneously in other centers. In most situations, IRBs should not approve a Phase 1 study that seeks to repeat other Phase 1 trials or is contemporaneous with other trials of the same agent.

2. Reject justifications for a Phase 1 protocol that are based on adjunctive elements unrelated to the research question. Arguments that the general quality of the medical care that they receive will be higher if they participate in a research study should never offset ethical compromises in research design.

3. Make clear the distinction between research and patient care. IRBs should reject in all written forms and should discourage, in the consenting dialog itself, the use of language that serves to blur the distinction between the enterprise of research and the activity of patient-centered care.

4. Require a commitment to eliminating misconceptions about risks and benefits. Specifically, potential subjects should be told that Phase 1 trials are designed to determine toxicity, that severe toxicity is a planned event for a subset of subjects, and that direct benefit is both not intended and extremely unlikely.

5. Require standardized wording in the consent document as follows:

Purpose: The purpose of this study is to find the highest dose of _____ that people can tolerate without getting extremely ill.

Risks: In this study, the dose of _____ will be increased until people get extremely sick. Because of the different dosing and how your body will tolerate the drug, it is impossible to predict the side effects that you personally will experience.

Benefits: This study was not designed and is not being done to treat your cancer. Based on prior experience, the chance that you will feel better or live longer as a result of participating in this study is almost zero. This study is being done in the hope that it will provide information that will improve the treatment of people in the future.

REFERENCE

Freedman, B. (1996). The ethical analysis of clinical trials: New lessons for and from cancer research. In H. Y. Vanderpool (Ed.), *The ethics of research involving human subjects: Facing the 21st century* (pp. 319–338). Frederick, MD: University Publishing Group.

The Health Insurance Portability and Accountability Act

ROBERT AMDUR AND ELIZABETH A. BANKERT

HIPAA for IRB Members

- IRB administrators and chairpersons should ensure that the study application is HIPAA compliant before it is presented to the IRB.
- HIPAA language requirements should be embedded within an institutional consent form template or added as an additional consent form.
- Because both items above will be completed prior to IRB member review, HIPAA requirements should not be discussed at every IRB meeting.

The acronym for the Health Insurance Portability and Accountability Act is HIPAA. The main goals of HIPAA are to enable employees who change jobs to obtain health insurance at a new job without being penalized for preexisting conditions (portability) and to decrease fraud and waste in Medicare billing (accountability). The law also includes an additional section of HIPAA-mandated standards for the storage and transmission of healthcare information in certain situations.

In response to the HIPAA mandate, the HHS wrote federal regulations known as the Privacy Rule and the Security

Rule, effective April 2003 and April 2005, respectively. These regulations require documentation to conduct research involving human subjects that was not needed prior to HIPAA.

References to HIPAA requirements that affect IRB review are included in the publications listed at the end of the chapter. Two areas for general informational purposes are (1) the addition of required elements in order to waive informed consent if protected health information is used and (2) specific information related to the use of subject data must be contained in the consent form. HIPAA introduces concepts including authorization, review preparatory to research, identified data, limited data set with a data use agreement, and business associate contracts to IRB administrative terminology. Some institutions have a privacy board to address HIPAA issues; other institutions have asked the IRB to take on the responsibilities. In either case, the requirements are complex and in general should not be part of an IRB meeting review. Rather, the requirements must be implemented via policies and procedures and transferred into consent form template language and information required in the IRB application.

References

Muhlbaier, L. H. (2006). Health insurance portability and accountability act and research. In E. Bankert & R. J. Amdur (Eds.), *Institutional review board: Management and function* (2nd ed.). Sudbury, MA: Jones and Bartlett.

National Institutes of Health. (2004). *Research repositories, databases, and the HIPAA privacy rule.* NIH publication No. 04-5489. Retrieved from http://privacyruleandresearch.nih.gov/research _repositories.asp

PART 4

RESOURCES

This portion of the handbook contains a listing of some of the resources available related to human subject research.

Ethical Codes

Belmont Report
National Commission for the Protection of Human
Subjects of Biomedical and Behavioral Research.
(1979). *Ethical principles and guidelines for the protection of human subjects of research.*
http://www.hhs.gov/ohrp/humansubjects/guidance/
belmont.htm

Nuremberg Code
http://www.hhs.gov/ohrp/references/nurcode.htm

World Medical Association Declaration of Helsinki
http://www.wma.net/en/30publications/10policies/
b3/index.html

U.S. Government Regulations

Biologic Products: General
21 Code of Federal Regulations Part 600
http://www.accessdata.fda.gov/scripts/cdrh/cfdocs/
cfCFR/CFRSearch.cfm

Department of Health and Human Services
Office of Human Research Protection (OHRP)
http://www.hhs.gov/ohrp

Financial Disclosure by Clinical Investigators
21 Code of Federal Regulations Part 54
http://www.fda.gov/RegulatoryInformation/
Guidances/ucm126832.htm

**Health Insurance Portability and Accountability
Act (HIPAA)**
http://aspe.hhs.gov/admnsimp

Investigational Device Exemptions
21 Code of Federal Regulations Part 812
http://www.accessdata.fda.gov/scripts/cdrh/cfdocs/
cfcfr/cfrsearch.cfm

Investigational New Drug Application
21 Code of Federal Regulations Part 312
http://www.accessdata.fda.gov/scripts/cdrh/cfdocs/
cfcfr/cfrsearch.cfm

Protection of Human Subjects
21 Code of Federal Regulations Part 50
http://www.accessdata.fda.gov/scripts/cdrh/cfdocs/
cfcfr/cfrsearch.cfm

Protection of Human Subjects
45 Code of Federal Regulations Part 46
http://www.hhs.gov/ohrp/humansubjects/
guidance/45cfr46.htm

Review Boards
21 Code of Federal Regulations Part 56
http://www.accessdata.fda.gov/scripts/cdrh/cfdocs/
cfcfr/cfrsearch.cfm

Revised Expedited Review Criteria (1998)
http://www.hhs.gov/ohrp/humansubjects/guidance/
expedited98.htm

U.S. Government Guidance/Resources

Bioethics Resource on the Web—National Institutes of Health
http://www.nih.gov/sigs/bioethics

FDA Clinical Trials/Human Subjects Protection
Information for Health Professionals
http://www.fda.gov/oc/oha/default.htm#clinical

FDA Information Sheets (1998 edition)
Guidance for Institutional Review Boards and
Clinical Investigators
http://www.fda.gov/oc/ohrt/irbs/default.htm

Food and Drug Administration (FDA)
http://www.fda.gov

National Human Genome Research Institute
Ethical, Legal and Social Implications of Human
Genetics Research
http://www.nhgri.nih.gov/ELSI

**National Reference Center for Bioethics
Literature—Kennedy Institute of Ethics**
http://bioethics.georgetown.edu

Office of Biotechnology Activities—NIH
http://www.nih.gov/od/oba/index.htm

Office for Human Research Protections (OHRP):
2009 Determination Letters
http://www.hhs.gov/ohrp/compliance/letters/
index.html

Office for Human Research Protections (OHRP):
Guidance Topics by Subject
http://www.hhs.gov/ohrp/policy/index.html#topics

Office for Human Research Protections (OHRP):
Guidebook
http://www.hhs.gov/ohrp/irb/irb_guidebook.htm

Office for Human Research Protections (OHRP):
Home
http://www.hhs.gov/ohrp

Office for Human Research Protections (OHRP):
OHRP Compliance Oversight Activities:
Determinations of Noncompliance
http://www.hhs.gov/ohrp/compliance/findings.pdf

Office of Research Integrity
http://ori.dhhs.gov

U.S. Department of Veterans Affairs PRIDE
Program for Research Integrity Development &
Education
http://www.research.va.gov/programs/pride/
default.cfm

International Guidelines

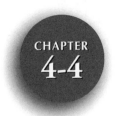

Canadian National Guidance Document
TriCouncil Policy Statement—Ethical Conduct for
Research Involving Humans
http://www.pre.ethics.gc.ca/eng/policy-politique/
initiatives/revised-revisee/Default/
National guidance document: TriCouncil Policy
Statement—Ethical Conduct for Research Involving
Humans
http://www.pre.ethics.gc.ca/pdf/eng/Revised%
20Draft%202nd%20Ed%20PDFs/Revised%20
Draft%202nd%20Edition%20TCPS_EN.pdf

**Council for International Organizations of Medical
Sciences (CIOMS)**
International Ethical Guidelines for Biomedical
Research
http://www.cioms.ch/index.html

International Committee on Harmonization (ICH)
Good Clinical Practice Guidelines
http://www.ich.org/LOB/media/MEDIA482.pdf

**National Council on Ethics in Human Research—
Canada**
http://www.ncehr-cnerh.org/english/home.php

World Health Organization
Department of Research Policy and Cooperation
http://www.who.int/rpc/en

Books

Bankert, E., & Amdur, R. J. (Eds.). (2006). *Institutional review board: Management and function* (2nd ed.). Sudbury, MA: Jones and Bartlett.

Beauchamp, T. L, & Childress, J. F. (1994). *Principles of biomedical ethics*, (4th ed.). New York: Oxford University Press, 1994.

Beauchamp, T. L., Faden, R. R., Wallace, R. J., Jr., & Walters, L. (Eds.). (1982). *Ethical issues in social science research*. Baltimore: Johns Hopkins University Press.

Beecher, H. K. (1970). *Research and the individual: Human studies*. Boston: Little, Brown.

Brody, B. A. (1998). *The ethics of biomedical research: An international perspective*. New York: Oxford University Press.

Dunn, C., & Chadwick, G. (1999). *Protecting study volunteers in research: A manual for investigative sites*. Boston: Center Watch.

Faden, R. (Ed.). (1996). *The human radiation experiments*. New York: Oxford University Press.

Faden, R. R., & Beauchamp, T. L. (1986). *A history of theory of informed consent*. New York: Oxford University Press.

Freund, P. A. (Ed.). (1970). *Experimentation with human subjects*. New York: George Braziller.

Jonsen, A. R, Veatch, R. M., & Walters, L. (1998). *Source book in bioethics: A documentary history*. Washington, DC: Georgetown University Press.

Katz, J., with the assistance of Alexander Morgan Capron and Eleanor Swift Glass. (1972). *Experimentation with human beings: The authority of the investigator, subject, professions, and state in the human experimentation process*. New York: Russell Sage Foundation.

Levine, R. J. (1988). *The ethics and regulation of clinical research* (2nd ed.). New Haven, CT: Yale University Press.

Penslar, R. L. (1995). *Research ethics: Cases and materials*. Bloomington: Indiana University Press.

Protecting human research subjects: Institutional review board guidebook. (1993). Bethesda, MD: Office for Protection from Research Risks.

Russell-Einhorn, M. (Ed.). (2000). *IRB reference book.* Washington, DC: Price Waterhouse Coopers, LLP.

Sieber, J. E. (Ed.). (1982). *The ethics of social research: Fieldwork, regulation, and publication.* New York: Springer-Verlag.

Sieber, J. E. (Ed.). (1982). *The ethics of social research: Surveys and experiments.* New York: Springer-Verlag.

Sieber, J. E. (1992). *Planning ethically responsible research: A guide for students and internal review boards.* Applied Social Research Methods Series, vol. 31. Newbury Park, CA: Sage Publications.

Sugarman, J., Mastroianni, A., & Kahn, J. (1998). *Ethics of research with human subjects: Selected policies and references.* Frederick, MD: University Publishing Group.

Vanderpool, H. Y. (1996). *The ethics of research involving human subjects.* Frederick, MD: University Publishing Group.

Veatch, R. M. (1989). *Medical ethics.* Sudbury, MA: Jones and Bartlett.

Periodicals and the IRB Forum

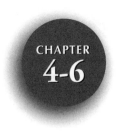

Bulletin of Medical Ethics
http://www.rsmpress.co.uk/bme.htm

The Hastings Center
http://www.thehastingscenter.org/Publications/HCR/
Default.aspx

Human Research Report
http://www.humansubjects.com

The IRB Forum (previously MCWIRB)
The IRB Forum (previously called MCWIRB) promotes the discussion of ethical, regulatory, and policy concerns with human subjects research.
http://www.irbforum.org

Journal of Empirical Research on Human Research Ethics
http://www.csueastbay.edu/JERHRE

Kennedy Institute of Ethics Journal
http://muse.jhu.edu/journals/ken

PRIM&R Newsletter
Public Responsibility in Medicine & Research
http://www.primr.org

Report on Research Compliance
http://www.reportonresearchcompliance.com

Research Practitioner
http://store.centerwatch.com/p-118-research-practitioner.aspx

Selected Publications

Fost, N., & Levine, R. J. (2007). The dysregulation of human subjects research. *Journal of the American Medical Association, 298*(18), 2196–2198.

Grady, C., & Levine, R. J. (2007). Commentary 13.2: Shared responsibilities for treatment in the South African phase 1 HIV preventive vaccine trials. In J. V. Lavery, C. Grady, E. R. Wahl, & E. J. Emanuel (Eds.), *Ethical issues in international biomedical research: A case book* (pp. 225–232). New York: Oxford University Press.

Kass, N., Pronovost, P. J., Sugarman, J., Goeschel, C. A., Lubomski, L. H., & Faden, R. (2008). Controversy and quality improvement: lingering questions about ethics, oversight and patient safety research. *The Joint Commission Journal on Quality and Patient Safety, 34*, 349–353.

Levine, R. J. (2008). The nature, scope and justification of clinical research: What is research? Who is a subject? In E. J. Emanuel, C. Grady, R. A. Crouch, R. Lie, F. Miller, & D. Wendler (Eds.), *The Oxford textbook of clinical research ethics* (pp. 211–221). Oxford, England: Oxford University Press.

Levine, R. J. (2008). Research involving adolescents as subjects: Ethical considerations. *Annals of the New York Academy of Sciences, 1135*(1), 280–286.

Levine, R. J. (2009). On the relations between scientists and journalists: Reflections by an ethicist. In P. C. Snyder, L. C. Mayes, & D. D. Spencer (Eds.), *Science and the media: Delgado's brave bulls and the ethics of scientific disclosure* (p. 153). Amsterdam, The Netherlands: Academic Press (Elsevier).

Levine, R. J. (in press). The institutional review board. In S. S. Coughlin & T. L. Beauchamp (Eds.), *Ethics in epidemiology* (2nd ed., pp. 257–273). New York: Oxford University Press.

Mathews, D. J., Sugarman, J., Bok, H., Blass, D. M., Coyle, J. T., Duggan, P., et al. (2008). Cell-based interventions for neurologic conditions: Ethical challenges for early human trials. *Neurology, 71,* 1–6.

Weinfurt, K. P., Hall, M. A., Dinan, M. A., DePuy, V., Friedman, J. Y., Allsbrook, J. S., et al. (2008). Effects of disclosing financial interests on attitudes toward clinical research. *J Gen Intern Med 23,* 860–866.

Organizations

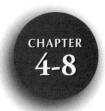

CHAPTER 4-8

American Society of Law, Medicine, and Ethics (ASLME)
http://www.aslme.org

CenterWatch Clinical Trials
http://www.centerwatch.com

Drug Information Association (DIA)
http://www.diahome.org

National Association of IRB Managers (NIAM)
http://www.naim.org

Public Responsibility in Medicine and Research (PRIM&R)
http://www.primr.org

Index